# Sacred Medicine Cupboard

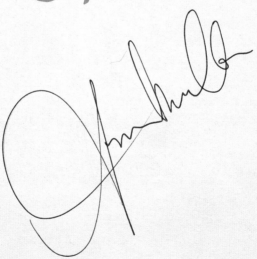

OTHER BOOKS BY ANNI DAULTER

*Sacred Pregnancy*
*Organically Raised*
*Ice Pop Joy*
*The Organic Family Cookbook*
*Naturally Fun Parties for Kids*
*Bountiful Baby Purees*
*Sacred Motherhood*
*Coming Soon: Sacred Relationship*

# Sacred Medicine Cupboard

## A Holistic Guide and Journal
## for Caring for Your Family Naturally

ANNI DAULTER,
JESSICA BOOTH,
AND
JESSICA SMITHSON

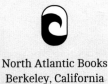

North Atlantic Books
Berkeley, California

Published by
North Atlantic Books
Berkeley, California

Cover photo by Heidi Marie Wagstaff,
Styling by Anni Daulter at Little Oyster
Cover design by Claudia Smelser
Interior design by Jasmine Hromjak and Claudia Smelser

Printed in the United States of America

MEDICAL DISCLAIMER: The following information is intended for general information purposes only. Individuals should always see their health care provider before administering any suggestions made in this book. Any application of the material set forth in the following pages is at the reader's discretion and is his or her sole responsibility.

*Sacred Medicine Cupboard: A Holistic Guide and Journal for Caring for Your Family Naturally* is sponsored and published by the Society for the Study of Native Arts and Sciences (dba North Atlantic Books), an educational nonprofit based in Berkeley, California, that collaborates with partners to develop cross-cultural perspectives, nurture holistic views of art, science, the humanities, and healing, and seed personal and global transformation by publishing work on the relationship of body, spirit, and nature.

North Atlantic Books' publications are available through most bookstores. For further information, visit our website at www.northatlanticbooks.com or call 800-733-3000.

LIBRARY OF CONGRESS CATALOGING-IN-PUBLICATION DATA

Names: Daulter, Anni, author. | Booth, Jessica, 1976– author. | Smithson, Jessica, 1976– author.
Title: Sacred medicine cupboard: a holistic guide and journal for caring for your family naturally / Anni Daulter, Jessica Booth, Jessica Smithson.
Description: Berkeley, California: North Atlantic Books [2016]
Identifiers: LCCN 2016019366 (print) | LCCN 2016022273 (ebook) | ISBN 9781623170684 (paperback) | ISBN 9781623170691 (ebook)
Subjects: LCSH: Naturopathy—Popular works. | Alternative medicine—Popular works. | Self-care, Health—Popular works | BISAC: HEALTH & FITNESS / Naturopathy. | FAMILY & RELATIONSHIPS / Parenting / General.
Classification: LCC RZ440 .D383 2016 (print) | LCC RZ440 (ebook) | DDC 615.5/35—dc23
LC record available at https://lccn.loc.gov/2016019366

1 2 3 4 5 6 7 8 9 Versa 22 21 20 19 18 17

# 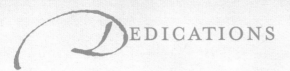EDICATIONS

To every soul who picks up this book, may you
see, feel, and experience your own medicine.
May you walk in balance with Mother Earth
as you flow through all of the transitions and
seasons of your life.
To my husband, Tim, for helping me always
strive to live in Divine Mind. And to my
children, Zoe, Lotus, Bodhi, and River, may
you all live in right relationship with the world
as you dance through every day.

—ANNI DAULTER

To all sweet souls on their healing path, may
this book bring a little light, joy, and inspiration
to your journey. To my husband, Leigh, who
held down the fort with humor and grace so I
could live my dream and write this book. To my
children, Eden and Rai, may you always hold
your wonder and divinity in your hearts as you
go through life.

—JESSICA BOOTH

To the amazing people who saw me even when I could not see myself, I am forever grateful. To my family, blood and chosen, who are more amazing than I have adequate words for, thank you for your love, support, wisdom, laughter, and endless inspiration. To everyone else, I hope this journey inspires you to find your medicine and feed your soul.

—JESSICA SMITHSON

# CONTENTS

# 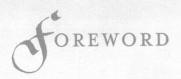OREWORD

You are a seeker. You have likely opened these pages looking for a path to the life that is calling you from the inside out. Sometimes this call comes as a yearning for what we know is possible but have not yet seen. Sometimes it comes from an innate guiding wisdom attuning us to what makes us more alive. Other times, we are hunting for deeper meaning to heal our sorrows, losses, and betrayals.

If you are a parent, you may be seeking this for the sake of your young ones, aligning your highest hopes with your greatest actions so that they can have the life you dream for them. Not only do I honor your journey that brings us together here; I also recognize our need for company, for teachings, for caring as kindred spirits.

Do you know that you are holding not only a book but a portal which, when used well, can bring you a plethora of choices and some entirely new landscapes to build your life upon, if you are inspired to take action? Only you, however, can be the medicine, the answer. Only you can leave your unique legacy and connect your heart with the great awakening that is calling us all. If you are not sure how powerful such a portal can be, then I would like to share my personal story with you.

I was visited by the Sacred in a mystical dream when I was eighteen years old, and the message I received guides my life even now, though I rarely share it. My dream awakened and anchored in me one of my deepest longings, and the belief that it is possible to find what you are seeking because in many ways what you yearn for most is also seeking you.

This epic vision began by knowing that on this particular day I would die. At first I acted heroically to escape all perils in order to survive. When sunset came, I stood triumphantly under the blue sky, believing I had survived the odds. This is when dark thunderclouds rose from the horizon, moving with uncanny speed like time-lapse photography, and aimed solely in my direction. One single stroke of lightning flashed, cracking my bones with a boom that I can still hear. Yet my life did not end here. My sister came running and held my body, a mere shell now in her arms as she wept. I found myself hovering above her, wanting to comfort her but to no avail. This is when I noticed that there was an angel spirit by my side. She told me that she was here to be my guide, and that if I would travel with her she would show me the seven doorways of life. Before you get your hopes up, I am only able to tell you about two of these—the first and the last.

In the first door, shrouded in darkness, were souls wandering without consciousness in brown, hooded robes. What was alarming is that they did not notice one another, least of all themselves, even when they bumped against each other in the dark. They lacked any awareness of interconnectedness, and witnessing this brought deep sorrow.

The last doorway was a far contrast from the first. The door itself was an arbor covered in leaves, ornate veils, and flowers, and when you entered you were embraced by music, the beauty of nature, unbelievable fragrances, colors, and people lying in groups on beds of green moss, and dancing freely in the waterfalls and streams. Entering, I beheld women and men talking together with more love, intimacy, and communion than I had ever seen. In cuddle-piles and with direct eye gazes, they were captivated in deep conversation and laughter. They seemed to easily hold complex, intimate emotions with compassion and kindness.

Children were playing among them, fed and tenderly cared for by their collective devotion. Everyone was respected. My heart was so moved that even now, as I write these words, tears come to my eyes. I wanted this authentic relationship with self and others, and this world of peace. As a teenage single parent to a one-year-old, I had little support; never before had I witnessed such a scene in my waking life. How could I get there? Was it really possible, or only a dream vision? The spirit woman assured me that one day this doorway would be mine to enter if I walked the path I was presently on with continued love, courage, and commitment. She was right.

Her words lit a promise in my heart. With this encouragement, each and every day since, I continue to seek all the wisdom I can find for my family and myself, promising to heal my heart with others even if it means confronting the darkest shadows in myself and humanity. Learning about the herbs, plants, and ceremonies as medicine, how to build community, how to get clear with others when there is conflict, how to walk with integrity, how to facilitate deep transformational work and initiations, and bringing in new paradigms such as the grassroots Red Tent Temple Movement and Building the Sisterhood Bridge, became some of my life's work.

With brave souls and change-makers, I became a trailblazer, a pioneer, while also drawing from ancient wisdom and from the Earth herself as my mother. This last door did indeed become mine to live from, and here is where I learned that what you cannot yet see can be brought into existence. It means grounding what you most want into form, through each choice and action we take in relationship to one another and ourselves.

Profound connections and stories beyond the telling are how I came to meet each of these beloved women authors—Anni, Jessica B., and Jessica S.—as far away as magical Cae Mabon in Wales to walking the Tor in Glastonbury to the beginnings of the Sacred Pregnancy Movement. You are the one they write for, hold intention for, the one who keeps their hearts burning bright. One of their deepest desires is to put medicine—your own—into your hands, the medicine that you are holding now in *Sacred Medicine Cupboard*.

What is here for you, if you choose to embark on it, is a way to enter. It is not the answer; instead, it is a portal. Like the doorway in my dream, *Sacred Medicine Cupboard* stands for what is possible if you want a healthy, whole, and holistic life. Words are words, and information is only information. A recipe is only words if it is never cooked. However, when you choose to follow the mystical path these authors describe, it can become your sojourn, page by page, action by action, season by season, as you become all the while more confident and sure of beauty, magic, and healing. The door is often closer than we know. May you enter and be blessed.

—ALISA STARKWEATHER,
FOUNDER OF THE RED TENT TEMPLE MOVEMENT

# 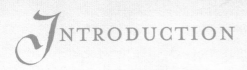NTRODUCTION

Welcome, friends, to your *Sacred Medicine Cupboard.* This book is an offering of wellness from our hearts to yours.

A few tenets hold this work in place. The first is that medicine belongs to everyone. It is your birthright—designed perfectly into your cells—to strive for health. We firmly believe that if you have the right tools and enough time, you can achieve thriving vitality.

The second guiding principle is that medicine is your innate wisdom, and that all living energies contain medicine to help us heal and thrive. Plants, crystals, animals, herbs, chakras, oils, essences, spirit guides, global and ancestral traditions—all have offerings to help us heal and to live a life of spiritual mastery.

One of the most profound medicines comes from right inside you. You have inhabited your body from the very first moment of cell division; you know yourself better than anyone else. This means your own experience of yourself is the most valid. Listen to your body and soul as you take this journey; they are your best and most reliable guide.

Finally, as you become the smith of your own wellness, we invite you to roll up your sleeves and fan the flames of wonder, magic, conjuring, inventing, and play. This book is a celebration of the beauty of these relationships, and an exploration of how they work for you. Take from it what resonates with you, play with what is new, and release the things that don't work for you.

Those of us who are parents or caregivers have a duty to be of service, and give care to our children and our wards. For the most part, we do it without thinking—we are caring, loving, and nurturing to those in our family. But how many of us have the skills we need to treat minor illnesses at home? How many of us are confident in talking about emotional challenges, or in creating a rich and varied landscape for spiritual experience with our families? Do we know what makes us happy and healthy on all levels? And how do we nurture those positive practices in our children?

*Sacred Medicine Cupboard* is a toolkit with answers to these varied and often complicated questions. Caregiving can be relaxed, fun, and even creative. One of the best gifts we can give to our children is gently supporting them in ownership of their own health and well-being. The soul challenges, herbal conjurings and crafty projects we invite you to explore in this book can, for the most part, be enjoyed by your whole family. You can share the intention and love in crafting these medicines and practices together. Teach each other what health means for all of you, living in your family and larger community.

## A note on wildcrafting

Many of the ingredients we use in this book can be either wildcrafted or cultivated in the right season. Lavender, calendula, and rosemary are hardy, generous plants and fairly easy to look after. Other popular and easy-to-grow herbs are marigolds, mints, lemon balm, nettle, and roses. Do not be afraid to nurture these friends yourself—in your garden, on a windowsill, or in the wild. We invite you to start a small herbal garden so that you can harvest them from your own backyard. We return the generosity of the plant kingdom by being generous caretakers of nature ourselves.

When you are wildcrafting, please respect the plants. Invest in a good-quality field guide such as *North American Wildland Plants* by James Stubbendieck, Stephan L. Hatch, and L. M. Landholt, or *Edible Wild Plants: A North American Field Guide to Over 200 Natural Foods* by Thomas Elias and Peter Dykeman, to be sure you are collecting the right plants.

## BASIC RULES FOR HONORING NATURE

- Always ask the plant before you take anything from it.

- Tell the plant what you are using it for—especially if you are making medicine. Be clear about the job at hand.

- Please do not take all of the plant; for example, leave some elderberries for the birds and critters who depend on that sustenance during winter. And the plant itself needs seeds to grow its next generation.

- Always say "thank you" to the plants you harvest from, to keep in right relationship with nature and Mother Earth.

## SACRED CUPBOARD BASICS

Collecting some basic equipment before you start will make conjuring the recipes in this book much easier. This is not an exhaustive list of all the recipe ingredients in the book; rather, it contains the basics for a well-rounded Sacred Cupboard for making remedies at home.

*Basic Sacred Cupboard equipment*

- A Sacred Cupboard space
- Journal
- Pyrex measuring jug
- Kitchen scales
- Spoons
- Metal or glass mixing bowls
- Cheesecloth
- Mesh strainer
- Wooden stirring stick
- Eye protection
- Disposable gloves
- Crockpot

- Blender
- Selection of Mason jars, all sizes
- Selection of very small jars and pots to store small quantities
- Spritz bottles
- Small dropper bottles
- Twine scissors
- Hot-water bottle
- Cotton cloth squares
- Pretty labels
- Pens, paper, art supplies

## Basic Sacred Cupboard ingredients

- Dried rose petals
- Dried lavender flowers
- Dried lemon balm leaves
- Dried calendula flowers
- Dried nettle leaves
- Dried hibiscus flowers
- Dried jasmine flowers
- Powdered turmeric
- Powdered cinnamon
- Powdered ginger
- Aloe vera gel
- Vitamin E
- Beeswax pastilles
- Castor oil
- Activated charcoal
- Apple cider vinegar
- Baking soda
- Coconut oil
- Almond oil
- Olive oil
- Cocoa butter
- Shea butter
- Raw local honey
- Witch hazel
- Rosewater
- Rose oil
- Sweet orange essential oil
- Grapefruit essential oil
- Rosemary essential oil
- Lavender essential oil
- Rose geranium essential oil
- Lemon essential oil
- Peppermint essential oil
- Ginger essential oil
- Pine essential oil
- Cinnamon-leaf essential oil
- Cedar essential oil
- Clove essential oil
- Sandalwood essential oil
- Frankincense essential oil
- Benzoin essential oil
- Rose essential oil
- Self-heal flower essence
- Yarrow flower essence
- Labradorite essence
- Rose essence
- White lotus essence
- Pomegranate flower essence
- Snowdrop flower essence
- Red peony flower essence
- Rose quartz
- Clear quartz
- Citrine
- Labradorite

# A NOTE ON STERILIZING BOTTLES

When preparing the recipes in this book, it is important to store the products of your hard work in clean, sterile bottles. This protects your balms and potions from cross-contamination. Our favorite method is the oven method; however, boiling works just as well. We do not recommend using the dishwasher for sterilizing bottles that will contain body products, as the trace salts left in bottles from the detergent can cause skin irritation in some people.

## Oven method

1. **Wash the jars and bottles.** Use hot water and dish soap to thoroughly wash the jars and bottles you plan to sterilize. Make sure they are completely free of dried food and other debris. Wash the lids as well; they must be scrupulously clean.

2. **Heat oven to 225° F/140° C/120° C fan oven/Gas 1.** After you have washed the jars in hot, soapy water and rinsed them well, place them on a baking sheet and put them in the oven to dry completely for at least twenty minutes. If using Kilner jars, boil the rubber seals, as dry heat damages them.

## Boiling method

1. **Wash the jars and bottles.** Use hot water and dish soap to thoroughly wash the jars and bottles you plan to sterilize. Make sure they are completely free of dried food and other debris. Wash the lids as well; they must be scrupulously clean.

2. **Place equipment in a deep pot.** Put the jars and bottles upright in the pot. Arrange the lid rings around the jars and bottles. Fill the pot with water, to one inch above the tops of the jars and bottles.

3. **Boil the jars and bottles.** Bring the water to a full, rolling boil. If you are at an altitude under 1,000 feet, boil them for ten minutes. Add an additional minute for each additional 1,000 feet of elevation.

4.  **Use tongs to remove the equipment from the water.** One by one, remove the jars, bottles, and lids, and place them on a paper towel to dry. Be careful not to let the sterilized equipment touch anything except the clean paper towel.

## Disclaimer

Information in this book is based on research from the internet, books, articles, studies, and our personal life experience. Statements in this book have not necessarily been evaluated by the FDA or any medical institution, and should not be considered as medical advice. Nothing in the book is intended to diagnose, treat, cure, or prevent any illness or disease. For diagnosis or treatment, consult your primary-care provider.

When using herbs, always start with the smallest amount for the shortest period of time, and work up from there. Use herbs and remedies in moderation, and watch for allergic reactions. Stop using them if you have any concerns.

If you are taking any other medication, are suffering from a medical condition, and/or are at all concerned about any of the advice or ingredients, consult your doctor before using any of the information shared in this book.

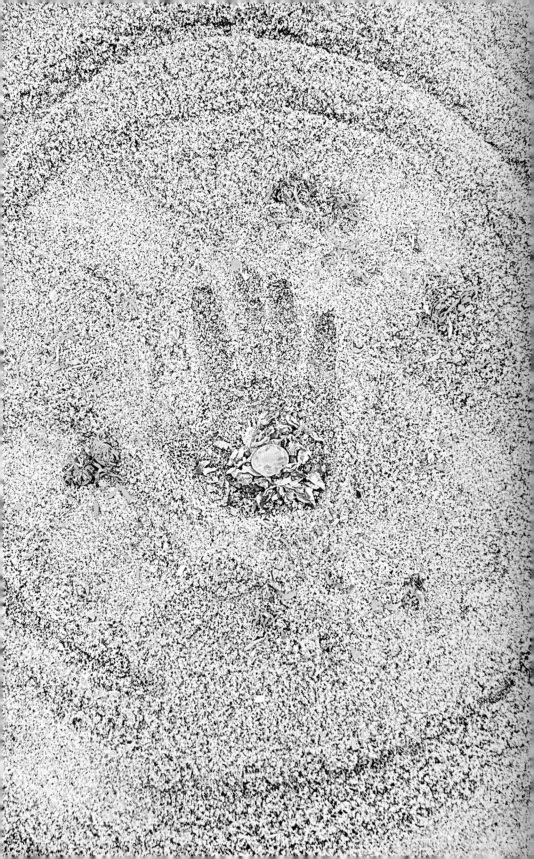

# PART ONE
# Spring

Arise, Earth Child, open your eyes,

behold the first stirrings of new life.

Drink the dew from the tips of the willow

and be reborn with the blissful elixir.

Bathe in the sweet trilling song of the bluebirds

and the whirring chirp of the ladybug.

Feed your heart with the secret whisperings of bees

calling love-sonnets to the flowers.

Awaken from your long winter's rest

and fall into the breath of life that is Spring.

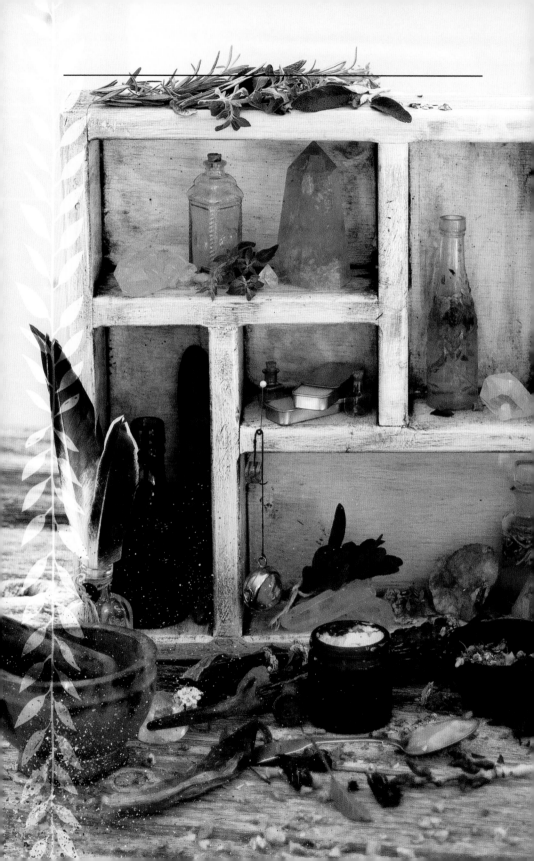

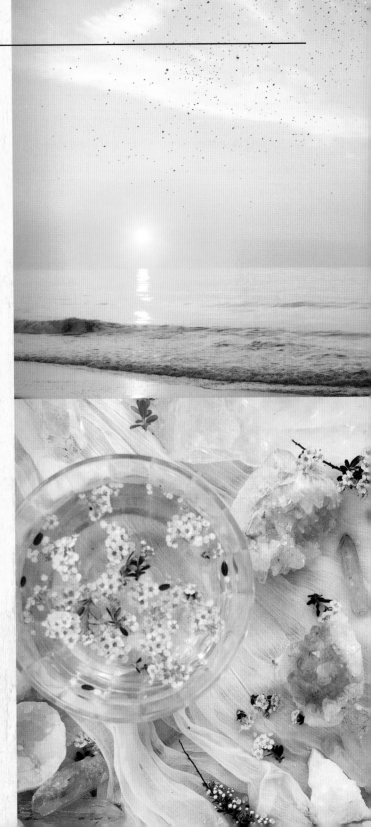

the dawn

*preparing the ground*

chapter I

*Spring is the season of birth, tender buds, opening, and fertility. It is time to pre-pare the rich soil of your whole self for health and healing. Arise with your entire being into the soft, subtle light of this first dawn. The aurora-glimmer of daybreak is both the beginning and the delicate moment of the in-between. Your potential is stretching its wings to soar into the unknown spaces of fresh starts and personal growth. Your limitless spirit beckons. Stand in the light, and say goodbye to the dark corners of your dreamland, willingly awakening your inner spark*

## FAMILY WELLNESS: *The Beginning*

Family wellness is a lifelong journey. Throughout this book, we will tread lightly on this path, walking with ease, patience, and unlimited trust. Let us start with the basic premise of one simple truth— your body naturally wants to heal. If you give it the right tools and the proper time, it will do its best to provide you with what you need.

In order to find your baseline condition and live in personal harmony, it is important to take an honest, non-judgmental look at where you are in this present moment. Let us start your walk toward living in balance by taking the time to make an objective tally of your and your family's physical, emotional, and spiritual state of being.

Begin a wellness journal, and list the following for each person in your family, marking the date so you can refresh your entry every twelve or thirteen weeks:

- **Physical information:** Height, weight, and waist circumference.
- **Make notes about:** The quality of your skin, hair, and nails, any medical conditions, food cravings (including preferences and dislikes), quality and quantity of sleep, energy throughout the day, and eating habits—including the when, how, and what of food consumption.
- **Body scan:** This can be done by simply checking in with each part of your body, taking note of any places of tightness, pain, weakness, or discomfort. Begin at the top of the head, and move down to the

eyes, ears, mouth, neck and throat, shoulders, upper back, arms, chest, ribs, stomach, lower back, lower stomach and pelvic bowl, hips, upper legs, knees, lower legs, ankles, and feet.

## SPIRITUAL APPLICATION: *Spiritual Well-being*

Spiritual health is the tonic to your body's physical strength, and is an integral part of holistic vitality. Exploring your spiritual well-being is a must-do first step. Let us start with a clear vision of how you truly live in this realm by using the fierce eyes of your spirit warrior and the discerning eyes of your inner hunter. In this way, you can track what you want in your life by following the trail to Divine Mind, the consciousness guided by pure love, with all of your senses. When you turn this potent gaze to your internal and external landscape, you can open your mind and heart to the truths that lie before you.

To begin clearing the way for the medicine that will bring health and vitality to your everyday life, keep the following acronym in mind: "SACRED."

## SOUL CHALLENGE: *Sacred*

Put SACRED into your life practice today. Write down the items in the acronym below, and after each one list one way that you are already practicing each quality, plus one way that you would like to practice it more.

**Soulfulness:** You have a space in your heart where you hold your soul's purpose and your life's legacy. Use this precious information as your guiding principle with each choice you make. Let it shape your course, and how you use your energy.

**Authenticity:** Show up with honesty and truth in every moment, and be kind to yourself when you do not.

**Connection:** Stay in tune with your body, thoughts, emotions, community, and family.

**Reverence:** Have deep and loving respect for your journey in life, bringing intention and mindfulness to each task.

**Enlightenment:** Lighten up and sparkle in the world! Listen to your heart's wisdom and knowing, taking into account the lessons you learn from your past, friends, family, and mentors.

**Dreaming:** Imagination is our creative ally; it is open throughout the night as we step into alternative consciousness. Be open to unfolding the magic of these other worlds.

## GLOBAL APOTHECARY: *Food is Medicine*

Most global medicinal traditions, from Ayurveda to Traditional Chinese Medicine to Mexican, treat food as medicine.[1, 2] Eating whole, organic, natural foods in a slow but quality manner is potent preventive medicine, and an important key to healing. There is no shortage of diet tips, tricks, and supposed must-do's in the world of getting fit—but the truth is that there is not one magic diet fad that will suit every person. So take it back to the basics!

*Plain and simple—healthy-eating basics*

- Stay away from processed foods full of chemicals and additives
- Eat whole, organic, fresh foods
- Chew your food well
- Avoid overindulgence
- Eat with intention and care

# Conjuring and Crafting

Assisting the health and well-being of your family will require an arsenal of knowledge pulled from every corner of your sacred home. Let's start by creating space for all the goodies you will make as you move through this book.

---

## CREATE A SACRED MEDICINE CUPBOARD

Recycle an old cabinet to store your remedies! This is a sacred space, and it needs your tender, loving care to bring it to life. You can do this together as a family, and as you clean, sand, paint, and decorate it, talk about your intentions. Tell stories, and whisper dreams into the wood. Share health and wellness wisdom with your children, and ask them what health feels like for them. For extra fun, you can add flower essences and essential oils to your cleaning products so the good vibrations soak into every cell.

(See Introduction for equipment and ingredients that you will want to gather to fill your basic Sacred Medicine Cupboard.)

Now that you have a space for medicinal treasures, let's make one! This cleaning powder is a perfect way to cleanse your space for the new journey you are about to embark upon.

---

## CLEANING POWDER AND SPELL

- 2 cups of baking soda
- 3 drops of cleansing flower essence, such as yarrow or white lotus
- 20 drops of your choice of the following essential oils: frankincense, sandalwood, rose, sweet orange

Assemble all your ingredients and your cauldron (a mixing bowl will do) and a wand (or a spoon works fine). Mix all the ingredients together with all of your love and intention. Hold your hands over the ingredients and say:

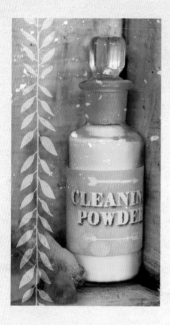

*Baking soda, flowers, pure heart too,*
*Bless my home, my heart, my body, and my spirit through.*
*Come together and clean for me.*
*Make my home negativity-free.*
*As above, so below. As it harm none, my will be done.*

Place the cleaning powder in a glass jar with a tight lid, label it "Cleaning Powder," and sprinkle it generously around your house. Then vacuum it up. Nothing is quite like a good sweep or vacuum for cleansing your space.

## MAKING A FLOWER ESSENCE

Try your hand at making a flower essence. The gift of the essences is the ability to teach us to connect to new vibrations; when we begin to resonate, anything can change. Choose any tree or flower growing in nature that calls to your heart—different plants have unique medicines.

### Sacred Medicine Flower Essence

- Glass bowl
- Piece of cheesecloth or strainer
- Pint-size Mason jar (to store mother essence)
- Pretty label

- I cup pure spring water or sacred water (water gathered from a holy, clean source)
- A live and thriving plant or flower from nature that wants to work with you
- I cup organic vodka or brandy.

The *sun method* is recommended for many essences, and is traditionally used for Dr. Bach's flower essences.

It is optimal to find a plant that is in full bloom and at the height of its energy. Prepare by meditating and asking to be called by a plant that wants to work with you. When you have heard the call of your plant, you need to ask it if it wants to be picked or not. This is a language that goes beyond words. Trust your instincts.

If the plant is okay with being picked, place the flower material in the bowl filled with pure spring or sacred water. Try to handle it as little as possible, because you don't want to add any of your own vibration to the essence. Some practitioners even use tweezers to lay the petals on the surface of the water; you can also use a leaf of the plant as a buffer between you and what you place in the bowl. Once you have done this, leave the bowl in the sun for several hours. You just need to feel when it is finished, as it varies from plant to plant. This guidance usually comes from the plant.

If the plant doesn't want to be picked, you will need to pour the water over the plant, catching it in a small bowl. You may want to do this several times, and then leave the bowl of water nestled next to the plant in the sun for several hours. Dr. Bach used to leave it for 3–4 hours but, again, you just need to feel when it is finished, as it varies from plant to plant.

When your essence is finished, strain the plant petals off using a strainer or cloth. The essence is then mixed with an equal amount of either vodka or brandy, and stored in a sterile glass jar. This is your mother tincture.

## Bottling your essence

*Our preferred method of sterilization is the boiling method—please see Introduction for details.*

## Stock

To make a stock essence from your mother tincture, fill a sterilized one-ounce bottle half-full with at least 40% ABV brandy or vodka. Add 2–7 drops (use your intuition) of your mother tincture, and fill it the rest of the way with pure spring water. This works out to about 50% preservative and 50% water. This is your stock bottle.

You can use this stock directly, or dilute it down to dosage if you are especially sensitive or if you will be giving it to sensitive people such as children or pregnant women, or to animals.

## Dosage dilutions

To make a bottle of dosage-strength flower essences, put 2–7 drops of your stock essence (or 2–7 drops of each essence if you are making a combination) into a one-ounce glass bottle ⅓-filled with brandy or vodka. Then fill the rest of the way with spring water. This now dosage dilution.

Instead of using brandy or vodka, you can also use vegetable glycerin. If you use glycerin, the contents will need to be used rapidly, as it has a shelf life of only about four weeks. Please refrigerate it, and be mindful not to touch your tongue to the pipette, as this may contaminate your essence with bacteria, and you will then need to throw it away.

Another way to reduce the amount of alcohol ingested is to put the flower essences in hot water and let it cool enough to drink; this helps the alcohol evaporate. This is a good option for those wanting to avoid alcohol altogether since, even if the dosage is made with vegetable glycerin, the mother essences always contain some alcohol.

With flower and gem essences, *less is more*. The changes that essences support can be deep and profound. It is better to proceed slowly and use at dosage strength, or dilute in water, unless you are well experienced with an essence. The only time to make an exception is during an acute situation, where signs and symptoms are high and sudden. This could be during labor, after a shock, or immediately after an accident or trauma, whether physical or emotional. In these cases, adding flower essences can be a great friend and complement to other first-aid methods.

## Pairings

- Crystal: Clear quartz. Place it in your medicine cupboard, and ask it to keep all your creations at a high, pure vibration.
- Flower Essence: Apple blossom essence. This essence is nourishing, cleansing, and supportive of your healing journey.
- Book: *The Mystic Cookfire: The Sacred Art of Creating Food to Nurture Friends and Family* by Veronika Sophia Robinson—a collection of soulful, healthy recipes.

# Journal

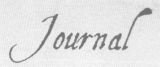

Take time to reflect on where you might be out of balance in your spiritual, emotional, and physical life, and note some positive changes you want to make:

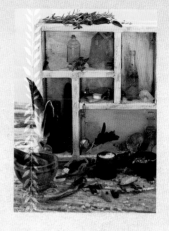

_____

_____

_____

_____

_____

_____

_____

_____

_____

_____

_____

_____

_____

_____

_____

_____

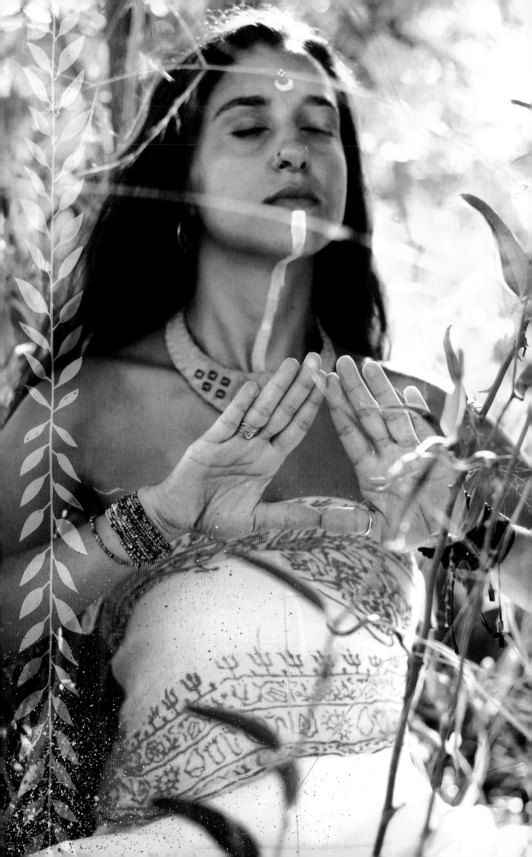

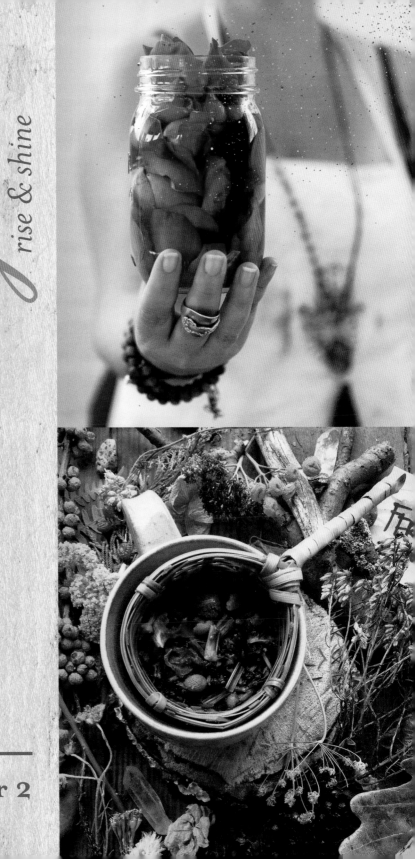

*awakening* rise & shine

chapter 2

*As Mother Nature bursts forth her glorious budding treasures at the onset of spring, so is this a time for your own personal awakening, to soul-stretch into a new form, flowing and bending with each passing season of your life. With the gentleness of new beginnings, use this space to take on the challenge of feeling into your own growth. Shedding skins of past narratives that no longer speak your truths will energetically invite "right relationship"—harmony with yourself and the totality of your environment, including nature and people. This work creates balance within your ever-changing story.*

## FAMILY WELLNESS: *Body and Soul Connection*

As the journey throughout this book truly gets underway, its important for you to deepen your understanding of just how tied your physical health is to your spiritual and mental bodies. This has been true from your first breath when you began to live out the *dharma,* or purpose, of this lifetime.

The stories you tell yourself about who you are directly affect your emotional well-being, which in turn affects the health of your physical body. We want you to be in harmonious balance within, so that you can live a strong and healthy life. Your body is your temple. It holds your soul with care, and so must you show it the respect of praying at its feet with reverence for how you speak to it, care for it, love it, and worship it.

## Prana, the Sanskrit word for "vital life"

*Prana* is the life-force that moves through us to keep our spirit bodies healthy and in tune. Understanding your *prana* can help you set intentions for a healthy internal landscape to bloom into its fullest potential. To keep your *prana* moving and in balance, practices need to be put into place. A healthy dose of meditation and yoga can keep you in balance, for sure, but we want to start with the basics.

*Setting intentions*

Everyone in your family can participate in and benefit from setting positive intentions for the day. Using Divine Mind—speaking heartfelt truths with love and compassion—is the best way to accomplish this daily practice. When you wake up in the morning, start with gratitude. Love and gratitude are the life-force of Divine Mind, the source in which its *prana* thrives and grows. Light a candle, and ask everyone in your home to say what they are grateful for. Then set your intention for the day—to have a love-filled day, to be love in every moment, to follow your heart-path, or to work on your heart's dream project, are all great examples of positive intentions for the day, and of feeding your spirit-body in order to enhance your physical and mental *prana*.

# SPIRITUAL APPLICATION: *Daily Practice*

A daily spiritual practice will help you stay in Divine Mind more often than not, and will offer up the medicine you may need to handle struggles and hurdles that may come your way.

The morning gratitude practice is a way to jump-start your spiritual engine, but to keep it running you will need to keep it fueled throughout the day. Affirmations are short, positive sayings that you can write down and place in various parts of your home or workplace. They remind you to stay in Divine Mind, come from love, be love, and soul-stretch when you need to. These little love-notes to yourself are helpful reminders, gifting your soul with internal peace throughout your daily routine.

# SOUL CHALLENGE: *Affirmations*

Give it a go! Write out five or ten positive affirmations and place them around your home and workplace. See how it makes you feel when you notice them throughout the day.

## GLOBAL APOTHECARY: *Break Up with Sugar*

What we put into our bodies can directly affect our mood, our spirit, and our mental bodies. Let's start by looking at sugar.

Studies show that foods that spike your blood sugar levels can have a very negative impact on your emotional health.[3, 4] While you may think that super-sugary treats are "feel-good" foods, they actually have the opposite effect on you, in both the short and long term.

It's very hard to cut sugar out of your diet when it's literally everywhere, but in the end it will result in a healthier mind, body, and spirit! Unlock your inner balance by kicking sugar, receiving into your body only foods that honor your temple and keep you in a high vibration.

## *Conjuring and Crafting*

### SACRED BODY TEMPLE TEA

*Makes four cups.*

Try this tea to replace sugar-laced drinks high in fructose and caffeine.

- ¼ cup rose petals
- 2 teaspoons cinnamon powder
- 1 cup hibiscus flowers
- ¼ cup jasmine flowers
- 2 drops orange essential oil
- 1 clear quartz crystal (to infuse the tea with its vibrational medicine)
- 1 rose quartz crystal (to infuse the tea with its vibrational medicine)

Put 4 cups of water, a clear quartz crystal, a rose quartz crystal, and the loose herbs into a pot. Bring to a boil, and let simmer for around 10–15 minutes to meld the flavors together. While your tea is simmering, say this prayer over it to raise the vibration of the tea:

*May this sacred tea nourish my body temple*
*with the intentions of raising my vibration, living in Divine Mind,*
*and honoring my spiritual, emotional, and physical bodies.*

After the tea has simmered, strain the loose herbs and crystals from the water, and store your tea in a large Mason jar to sip throughout the day.

## COLOR A YANTRA

A yantra is a geometric design, literally meaning *"a device that serves as a tool."* It is made with precision and delicate care to represent the body and its connection to the divine. This practice stems from Hindu traditions, and is like a prayer and offering to the gods that can help bring discipline and bal-

ance to your relationship with the divine. To get you started, you can find designs of yantras in adult coloring books, and online.

- Paper
- Ruler
- Colored pencils
- Pencil sharpener

Use a mandala-like design that you can find either in a coloring book or online, and try to recreate it on your own, adding colors to represent various chakras you may want to focus on. Keep your yantra in a sacred space in your home, to enhance your daily gratitude practice and meditations.

## TEA MANDALA

A mandala is a circular design used in Buddhist meditations on beauty and our relationship to infinity. It is effectively a visual prayer, offered up to the universe, that encompasses all of our relations and the never-ending cycle of life. Creating this Tea Mandala will be done with the same intention as a flower or sand mandala, but using different objects.

- Clear quartz crystals
- Feathers
- Cup of Sacred Body Temple Tea (above)
- Loose herbs

Gather your items and close your eyes, asking what the design should look like.

With delicate care, begin to create a mandala design by arranging your items, using your tea as the centerpiece of the meditation. Once your design feels complete, thank the universe for guiding you in this practice—and then disassemble it.

Taking it apart represents the impermanence of life and the ever-flowing gifts that change affords us.

## ROSE QUARTZ AND ROSE PETAL ELIXIR

Roses have one of the highest vibrations in nature; being around them instantly lifts us to a raised state of being. They are soothing, fragment, beautiful, and divine. This is a plant with a huge family, and she can be found everywhere people are. She grows both wild and cultivated. Roses are a true elixir for the heart and soul. Rose quartz adds a heart-opening and soothing note to the song of this elixir.

- I pint jar
- I cup organic vodka or liquor
- ½ cup pure spring water
- I rose quartz
- ½ cup raw local honey
- Enough fresh organic rose petals to fill the jar; if using dried, enough to fill ½ the jar
- 3 drops rose flower essence
- ⅛ cup aromatics of your choice—lemon, orange, grapefruit zest, or dried ginger
- I vanilla bean

Place your rose quartz in a glass with the spring water, and leave for 24 hours. Strain out the quartz and set water aside.

Pack your rose petals into the jar. Add vanilla and aromatics. Mix the honey with the vodka and water, and fill the jar with that mixture. Cover the top with thin fabric, plastic wrap, or a piece of waxed paper before tightening the lid. This keeps your elixir from corroding the lid and becoming contaminated. Shake well after closing securely.

Let sit for 4–6 weeks, shaking every few days. We like to make figure-eight patterns while shaking, and sing songs to the elixir about the medicine it is becoming. Strain it at the end of that time, and gift the herbal remains to your compost.

Use the elixir as you feel called to—topically, internally, spiritually. It really is magic.

*Pairings*

- Book: *Earthing: The Most Important Health Discovery Ever?* by Clinton Ober, Stephen T. Sinatra, MD, and Martin Zucker—explores the scientific foundation of why physical contact with the Earth is essential to well-being, and a great way to tune into your relationship with nature.

- Music: "Amrit Naam" by Bachan Kaur. The perfect partner for your creative explorations and the tea ceremony.

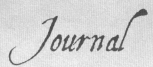

# Journal

List your daily affirmations here, and use this space to sketch your yantra meditation picture. You may also be called to navigate your relationship with your Divine Mind, and with barriers that may get in the way of living in your highest self throughout the day.

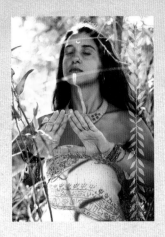

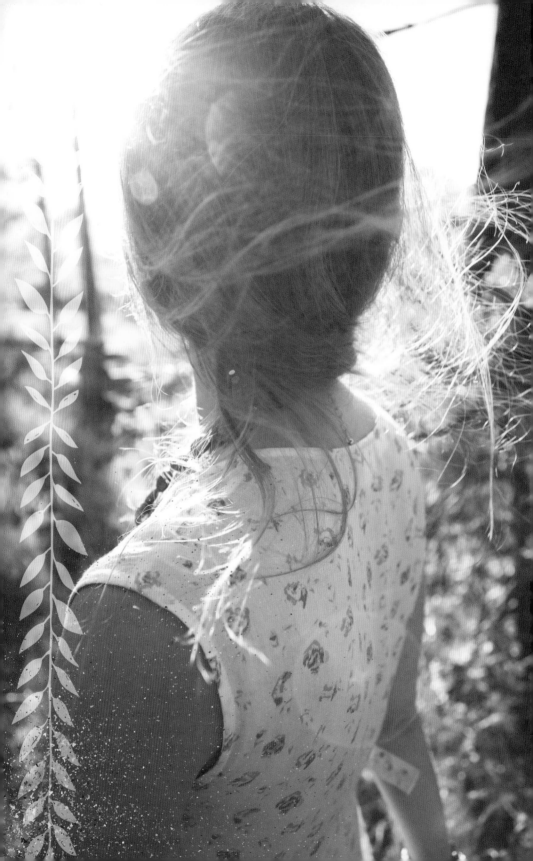

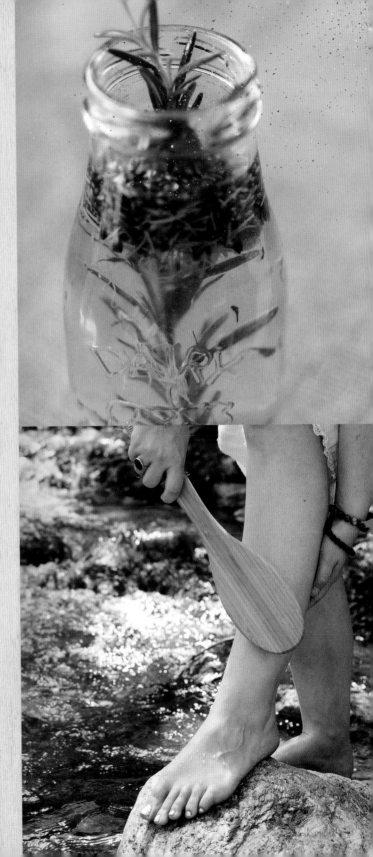

_spring equinox_

detoxing & cleansing

chapter 3

*Equinox, whether in spring or autumn, is a time of year when the light of the day is equal to the dark of the night. It is a moment where all life seems suspended in quintessential balance. As you evolve into your most divine being, pause in wonder: You have the spark of brilliance in you already. Your body is a microcosm of the Earth and the cosmos.*

*Ask yourself, from this vantage point, what do you thirst for? What can you cultivate to feed yourself, body and soul? What in your life needs pruning? You are the gardener of your precious dreams and of your blooming health. Each act of love and care is a seed well planted.*

## FAMILY WELLNESS: *Detoxing*

Spring is the time of growth and expansion in nature, and in you. In Traditional Chinese Medicine, it is the season associated with the liver and the gall bladder. This means that these organs naturally function at their peak during this season, and it is the perfect time of year to take extra steps to nourish them.

One primary function of your liver and gall bladder is to support detoxification of your blood. These days, our environment contains many more chemicals than ever before, from pesticides in food to plastics in the home to pharmaceuticals in the drinking water.[5, 6] You don't live in a bubble—and probably wouldn't want to! Instead, focus on supporting the body's natural ability to filter out these things.

*5 easy, gentle ways to begin detoxing as a family*

1. **Eat real food.** Reducing your consumption of processed food will easily eliminate many toxins from your body.

2. **Take a vacation from booze and coffee.** Reducing caffeine and alcohol removes common stressors to your liver, and gives your body a break.

3. **Invite in some green friends.**[7] Green smoothies, juices, and supplements such as chlorella, cilantro, and nori are great at clearing

out toxins. Start slow, with small quantities, and see how you feel.

4. **Light exercise,** such as rebounding or walking.

5. **Laughter**—it detoxes the heart and soul like nothing else!

Signs that your liver is processing toxins well include more energy, lighter periods, better sleep, even moods, and glowing skin.

## SPIRITUAL APPLICATION: *Integration and Release*

Life is a continuous flow of growth phases followed by journeys of integration and release. As you integrate new ideas, perceptions, and spiritual-development leaps, your old habits do not always make the cut. The scope of our lives is ever-changing, and it is okay to change your mind. It is even better to give yourself a break for not being born perfect. News flash, Baby—no one is! Spiritual growth is a spectrum, and requires patience and practice. Babies are not born with the ability to dance. No! They learn to wiggle after many careful steps, falls, and a lot of trial and error.

Give yourself permission to try on new ideas, allowing yourself to integrate what truly resonates for you. Do not be afraid to de-clutter your mind, throwing away outdated ways of thinking or being that no longer feel right, or no longer fit your spiritual narrative. Shed past behaviors and attitudes with gratitude in your heart, as these first bumpy steps will lead you down your heart-path in life.

## SOUL CHALLENGE: *De-Clutter*

Spring-clean more than just your body and your home: Find your "Holy NO!" and de-clutter your energy too. Using your Holy NO means you set boundaries consistent with your heart's purpose, and only agree to what serves you.

Use your Divine Mind, connect with your heart, and see if there is some way you are spending your precious time or energy that doesn't fit with your health-and-wellness goals. Then let go of it.

## GLOBAL APOTHECARY: *Dry-Brushing*

Dry-brushing is the practice of exfoliating the skin and unclogging the pores. It stems from many global traditions including Scandinavian and Asian medicine. It can stimulate the lymphatic system to aid in the removing of waste and toxins, and it also increases blood circulation—and feels invigorating.

All you need is a natural-bristle brush with a long enough handle to reach all parts of your body.

### How to dry-brush your skin

1. Dry-brushing is done before bathing, on your dry skin. Try soft, circular, upward motions followed by long, even strokes. Or simply use long strokes if that feels better.

2. Work from bottom to top, beginning at your feet and usually brushing in upwards movements in the direction of the heart – this motion and direction helps the lymphatic fluid drain from tissues, as lymph flows through the body towards the heart.

3. On your back, brush from the neck down to the lower back.

4. Be mindful and kind with delicate skin around the breasts and other tender areas.

5. If you have hot, inflamed areas, sores, sunburnt skin, skin cancer, open wounds, or seeping rashes, *do not brush these areas.*

6. When you are finished, shower well, rinsing all the dead skin flakes and impurities off your body.

7. Finish with a loving application of a body oil such as coconut.

### HERBAL LEMONADE

Herbal lemonade is a tea infusion mixed with a lemonade syrup to make a refreshing tonic. It is wonderful any time of year, but really shines in spring and summer. Lemons are healthy for your body, providing lots of vitamin C and nourishing the liver. Depending on what other herbs you choose, you are only adding to the goodness.

You can swap out the herbs below for any of your favorites. Other popular and delicious choices include lavender, rose petals, chamomile, mint, and hibiscus.

- 11 cups pure water
- 1 Tablespoon dried organic citrus peel (I love grapefruit for this)
- ¼ cup dried nettle
- ¾ cup dried lemon balm
- ¾ cup dried lemon verbena
- The zest and juice of 4 organic, unwaxed lemons
- ¼ cup (more or less, to taste) of sweetener; raw honey or maple syrup are great, but plain organic sugar is okay too—and it is okay to use less sugar

Boil 8½ cups of water, then turn off heat. Stir in the dry herbs and citrus peel. Cover well and leave until completely cool, or overnight. Strain herbs out and compost them. Reserve liquid infusion; this is your herbal tea base.

Place lemon zest and 2½ cups of water in small saucepan, and cover. Gently simmer over low heat for 3–5 min—do not overboil. Remove zest from the warm water and add the syrup or honey. Mix in the lemon juice and taste for the just-right sweet/sour balance; add more sweetener or lemon as needed. This is your lemonade base.

To serve, combine equal parts lemonade base, herbal tea base, and water. Feel free to adjust the quantities to suit your palate. This is pretty garnished with edible flowers or herbs and lemon slices. It can be stored in the fridge for up to 4 days.

## COCONUT MILK SHAMPOO

This easy, gentle cleansing shampoo is great for giving your hair a break from regular shampoo build-up. **Note:** This shampoo will not lather!

- ½ can full-fat pure coconut milk (without additives)
- 3 Tablespoons raw honey
- 3 Tablespoons aloe vera gel
- 3 Tablespoons argan oil
- 20 drops rosemary essential oil
- 20 drops orange essential oil
- 3 drops grapefruit flower essence

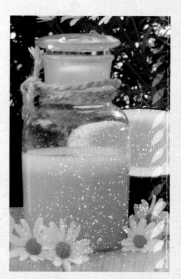

Whiz all the ingredients in a blender until smooth. Keep in a bottle and use in place of your regular shampoo. Massage into scalp and hair, and leave on for a few minutes before rinsing off.

## HERBAL VINEGAR HAIR RINSE

*This recipe is a gift from our dear friend Sarah Josey
from Golden Poppy Herbal Apothecary.*

- Pint-size Mason jar
- Plastic wrap
- Cheesecloth
- ¼ cup herbs of choice:

For **dark hair**—equal parts nettle and rosemary

For **light hair**—equal parts chamomile and calendula

For **red hair**—equal parts hibiscus and rose

- Apple cider vinegar

Place desired herbs in Mason jar. Cover herbs with apple cider vinegar to about one inch above the herbs. (You may need to add more vinegar after a couple of days, as it gets absorbed by the herbs, which is fine.) Cover the opening of the jar with plastic wrap (this prevents the vinegar from touching the metal jar lid and corroding it), and then seal the jar with the normal lid. Allow herbs to soak for 3 weeks minimum, shaking every so often.

When ready to use, strain out the herbs through the cheesecloth, being sure to squeeze out the liquid. Before your shower, place 1–2 Tablespoons of the infused vinegar into a nonbreakable cup that you can take into the shower. After you have washed your hair, dilute the vinegar in the cup with warm water. Slowly pour the diluted herbal vinegar over your hair, being sure to cover as much of it as possible, and working it in with your other hand at the same time. Allow vinegar to sit on your hair for 5 minutes. Rinse with cool water.

You're all done! The vinegar smell will fade as your hair dries, but you can always add a small amount of scented oil to your hair as a leave-in treatment.

*Pairings*

- Music: "Budding Trees" by Nahko and Medicine for the People—perfect inspiration for spring cleaning.

- Activity: *Seed-planting. This is the time to plant seeds—something sweet for your heart, something beautiful for your soul, and something sturdy for your roots.*

- Supplement: Amazing Grass—this powdered-greens supplement for adults and children mixes into smoothies with your milk of choice, for a tasty "milkshake" that helps cleanse the system and provides a powerful boost.

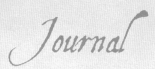

# Journal

What tender buds are you cultivating in your life now? What new perspectives are you integrating?

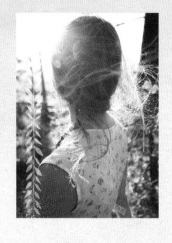

_____

_____

_____

_____

_____

_____

_____

_____

_____

_____

_____

_____

_____

_____

_____

_____

_____

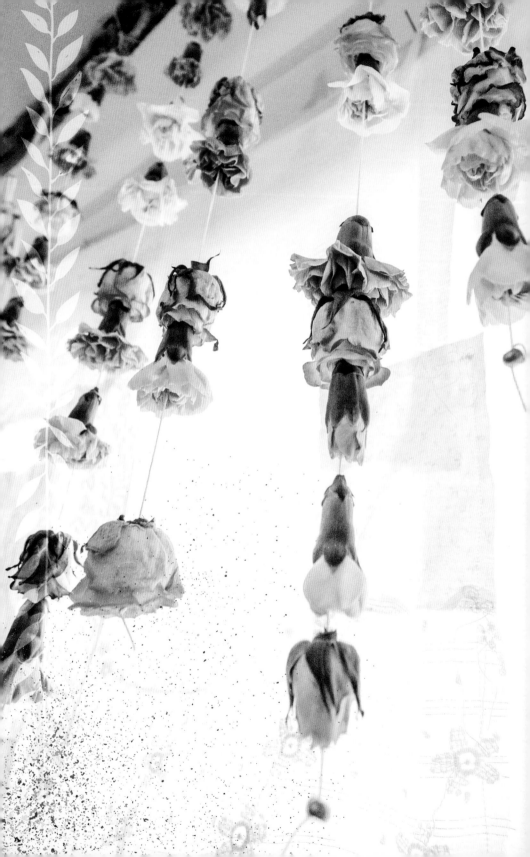

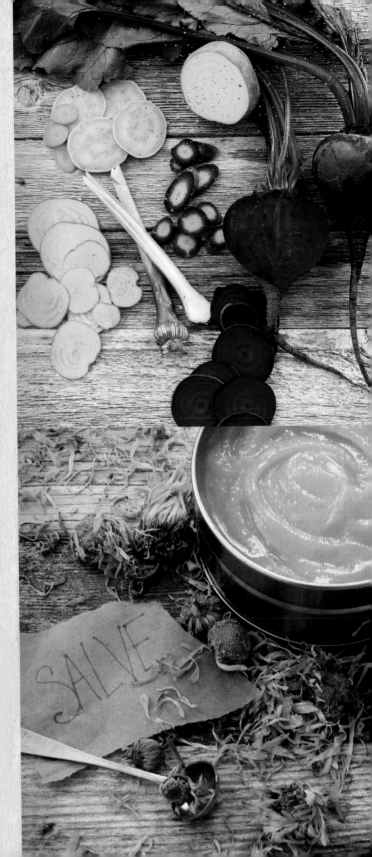

# the bud

*childhood blossoming*

## chapter 4

Children fall into every season of their lives with open eyes, tingling senses, and abundant curiosity. They are the promising young sprouts of the mature adults. Their days are full of adventures, discoveries, incredible creations, and rapid growth. Children are free to roam and experience everyday anew, unfettered by the gravity of adult stressors.

During this thrilling time, everything is possible, magic is real, and there are no expectations or preconceived ideas. Children believe that they can do anything and be anybody. Now is the time to nurture these tender buds with love, wholesome nutrition, and a sprinkling of inspiration.

## FAMILY WELLNESS: *Eat a Rainbow*

Make the most of your children's natural curiosity and creativity by introducing healthful dietary practices through the game of "rainbow eating." This is not the multi-colored world of processed foods, harmful dyes, or chemical additives; it is the rainbow of nature's candy, a plethora of whole foods bursting forth from Mother Earth herself.

Various colors of fruits and vegetables have unique vitamins and minerals that serve your body throughout each season.[8, 9] By eating a rainbow, i.e., a wide variety of colored vegetables and fruits, you are ensuring optimal health and vital longevity. When your family takes up this task of rainbow eating, aim for three to five different colors of real food on your plates at every meal. Let go of expectations of how much your family is consuming, and replace it with fun, experimentation, and play.

Here is a breakdown of the nutrients found in various colored foods, and some examples of vibrant, real foods.

### Red-colored foods

*Amazing for heart health and antioxidant support.*
**Nutrients:** Lycopene

**Foods:** Strawberries, beets, cherries, blood oranges, pomegranates, tomatoes, red bell peppers, red onions, red apples

## Blue/purple-colored foods

*Work wonders for memory, and slow down the aging process.*
**Nutrients:** Antioxidants

**Foods:** Eggplants, red cabbages, blueberries, blackberries, grapes, plums, elderberries, pomegranates, raisins

## Green-colored foods

*Support healthy cells and optimal body function.*
**Nutrients:** Chlorophyll

**Foods:** Broccoli, cabbage, bok choy, Brussels sprouts, kiwis, green grapes, avocados, spinach and other leafy greens

## Yellow/orange-colored foods

*Aid digestion and support the nervous system.*
**Nutrients:** High vitamin C

**Foods:** Apricots, butternut squash, cantaloupes, papayas, carrots, pumpkin, pineapples, peaches, oranges, sweet potatoes

## White-colored foods

*Assist with bone health and circulation.*
**Nutrients:** Phytochemicals and potassium

**Foods:** Cauliflower, garlic, mushrooms, onions, potatoes, pears, bananas

## SPIRITUAL APPLICATION: *Children as Open Beings*

Children are energetic sponges, soaking up information, emotions, and nuances from their environment. This makes it far easier to live as a spirit being than mired in the mundane adult physical world. Bruce Lipton says this process of being an open receptacle—like a new computer with unlimited memory—goes on intensely for the first seven years of life.[10]

Looking even further, children process and filter all that gets poured into their experiential wells. In these early years, children are learning with all their senses, making every interaction tangible and meaningful. Young children start with observation and imitation, which directly impacts their common understanding of life in the family and ultimately in the larger community.

Knowing this offers you the conscious opportunity to be a loving first example for your children. Allowing them to shine their spirit selves into the world, and explore every facet of their huge imaginations, may offer them a deep and profound spiritual base for growing their physical bodies and becoming more grounded in the world around them.

## SOUL CHALLENGE: *Imagination*

Use the "doodle game" to play with the idea that anything is possible. One person closes his eyes and draws a squiggle on a piece paper. The next person, with her eyes open, gets to turn the squiggle into a picture. This game can also be played as team.

## GLOBAL APOTHECARY: *Plant Spirit Medicine*

One of the key principles in the tradition of Plant Spirit Medicine is the understanding that the plants that grow in our local environment have the most potent medicine for us.[11, 12] For example, if you find you have an abundance of nettles growing in your garden—why not try nettle soup? The plants want to serve you and your family, and can be among your best allies when seeking health and wellness. When you take care of them, they in turn will take care of you. Plants that thrive without any intervention are especially potent in their medicine gifts.

# Conjuring and Crafting

## JEWELED RICE

This is a fun and colorful dish on its own, or as a side dish. It is tried-and-true, and tested by the experts—our kiddos! Our children love this healthy recipe, and would eat it every day. Add an additional spiritual component to the recipe by offering up a blessing over your dish—that it may nourish your family with all of the love you are pouring into its creation!

- 1 cup jasmine rice
- 1 Tablespoon coconut oil
- 1 teaspoon turmeric
- 1 teaspoon fresh-ground black pepper
- 1 pinch saffron
- 1 can coconut milk (7 ounces)
- 1 cup stock (chicken or veggie)
- ½ carrot
- ½ purple pepper
- ½ zucchini
- ¼ cup corn (non-GMO)
- ¼ cup peas
- ¼ cup pomegranate seeds
- 1 handful fresh coriander leaf

Place oil, turmeric, and black pepper in the saucepan, and slowly heat to infuse the oil. Cooking turmeric in fat with black pepper makes the curcumin, the medicinal part, bio-available.[13] Add the rice, and stir until it's coated with the yellow oil. Add coconut milk, stock, and saffron, and bring to a boil. Once boiling, turn it down to simmer for 20 minutes.

While this is cooking, dice the carrot, pepper, and zucchini, and then add all the veggies to the simmering rice for the last 10 minutes.

Garnish with pomegranate seeds and coriander leaf. Enjoy this with your family.

---

## INFUSED OILS OF CALENDULA, LAVENDER, AND CHAMOMILE

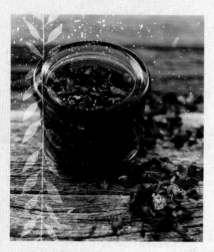

One part of the exuberance of childhood is weathering bumps and bruises. Here is a lovely healing salve made up of flowers full of medicinal properties. Thanks, nature! Try to pick plants that grow in your native environment, for extra potency. Feel free to add dried rose petals to this recipe for their fragrance and uplifting qualities.

**Calendula** *(Calendula officinalis)*—astringent, anti-inflammatory, and great for wound-healing[14]

**Lavender** *(Lavandula officinalis)*—lowers stress; antibacterial and pain-relieving[15]

**Chamomile** *(Matricaria chamomilla)*—reduces inflammation; antispasmodic and calming[16]

- 8-ounce glass jar (dark-amber color is best)
- Cheesecloth or strainer
- Wooden stick for stirring
- 8 ounces dried flowers—choose from calendula, lavender, or chamomile
- 8 ounces carrier oil (olive or almond)

- 2 teaspoons vitamin E oil as a preservative

You can combine the herbs here to make one oil—or make three separate oils, which gives you the freedom to really personalize the recipe.

Add dried flowers to the jar, and pack them down so the jar is full. You may need to add more than 8 ounces, once packed down. Add enough carrier oil into the jar to cover the flowers, stirring them with a wooden stick to release any air bubbles.

Cover the jar and leave it to infuse on a windowsill in the sun for 2–4 weeks. The longer you leave it, the more potent it will be. Give the oil a little turn and shake daily, making sure all the plant material is covered by oil.

When finished, strain flowers out and compost them. Add vitamin E oil to your infused oil, and store in a dark jar out of direct sunlight.

---

## SOOTHING SALVE

*Makes 4 jars.*

- Four 2-ounce jars
- I cup Infused Oil of Calendula, Lavender, and/or Chamomile (above)
- 3 Tablespoons beeswax
- I Tablespoon cocoa butter
- 20 drops lavender essential oil
- 10 drops rose geranium essential oil
- 3 drops of self-heal flower essence
- 5 teaspoons vitamin E oil, as a preservative

Heat the oil, beeswax, and butter in a double-boiler (or set a heatproof container on a pan of water on the stovetop) until liquefied. Remove from heat and allow it to cool a bit. Add the essential oils, flower essence, and vitamin E.

The texture of this salve can easily be adjusted. Before pouring your recipe into the containers, make a tester by placing a small scoop in the freezer for a minute to set up. Remove and check firmness. For a softer, more spreadable salve, add more oil. For a harder salve, add more beeswax. Once the consistency is to your liking, pour the salve into your jars and let it cool completely.

Use as needed for bumps and bruises.

## Pairings

- Book: *How to Eat a Rainbow: Magical Raw Vegan Recipes for Kids* by Ellie Bedford—a magical-themed recipe adventure.

- Reference: Plant identification guides for your local area—an indispensable reference for the budding herbalist.

# Journal

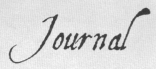

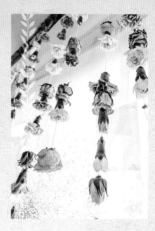

Sometimes the food we need to nourish us is not simply something to eat. It may be that we need to have our body, mind, emotions, or spirit fed in some other way. Many of us confuse this kind of message from the body, and head for the kitchen rather than looking for alternative sources of nourishment.

_____

_____

_____

_____

_____

_____

_____

_____

_____

_____

_____

_____

_____

_____

_____

_____

_____

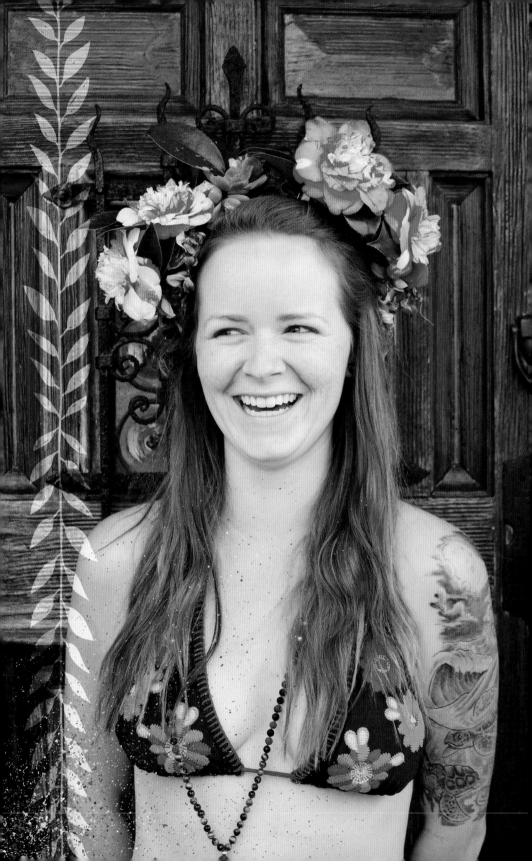

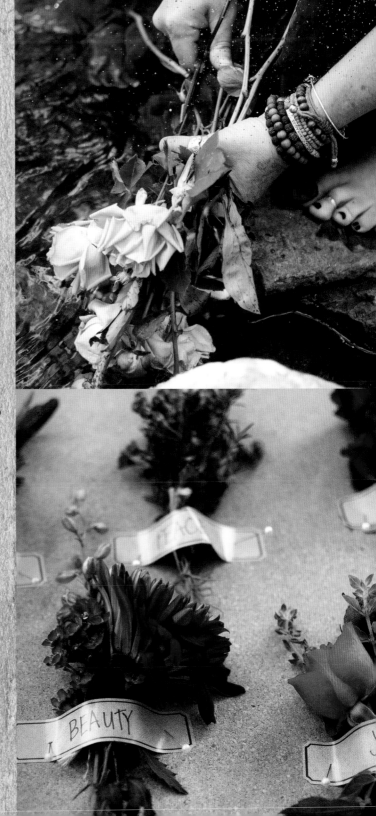

# blossom

*where flowers bloom, so does hope*

chapter 5

List other ways besides eating that you can "feed" your soul, spirit, and body:

*You stand peacefully in the enfolding tunnel of spring trees resplendent in blossom. Soft petals cling to your hair, and the scent of sweet nectar fills the air. You feel the call of the maiden, full of curiosity, innocence, and possibility.*

*Blossoming is a state of renewal and resurrection. It is a fragile threshold between becoming and undoing, between life and death. Blossoming is the sign of a plant completing a full life-cycle and beginning again—the cycle of birth and rebirth. You too have this capacity, this grace of beginnings within endings.*

## FAMILY WELLNESS: *First Aid 101*

First aid is what helps bring you fully back into your body after a shock. Think about when you put your hands on a child's ouchy and tell them everything is going to be okay. Remember a time that you hugged a loved one and said, "I'm here—you are safe." This simple touch, paired with eye contact and gentle words, is extremely potent healing magic. It is all the power of intention and action, effectively influencing actual experience. It may not cure a serious injury, but this heartfelt presence offers real, tangible succor in times of distress.

First aid in a serious emergency can be life-saving, and it is worth taking a class to feel confident in the hands-on techniques that are taught. This is your body, and knowing the basics of what can keep you alive in unexpected circumstances is a handy tool for any body to have!

Here are some basics: Children age six and under can be taught to call for help and to hold the hand of someone in need. Older children can practice the beginning assessment (see "DRS ABC" below) and bandaging limbs—always a popular game. Go ahead and have fun role-playing these skills with your children, so they can put practices into place with your loving guidance.

What is first aid? Well, the name says it all. It is the comfort you give first, before anyone else arrives. You may or may not be a fully trained doctor, but chances are you are qualified to give basic first aid.

The Red Cross has developed a super-easy memory aid—"**DRS ABC**":[17, 18]

**D** is for danger. If someone has been injured, it is because they were in a dangerous situation. Before rushing in to help, take a look around and make sure you are not putting yourself in danger too.

**R** is for response. Is the person responsive—do they answer when you call to them, or move when you touch them? You can ask simple questions such as, "What is your name? Can you see me?"

**S** is for shout for help. This means to call emergency services and ask for more people to support you both.

Now you can move into a basic assessment of the person—this is vital information to feed back to the emergency services.

**A** is for airway. If the person is unconscious, gently tilt their head back, lifting the chin to open the airway.

**B** is for breathing. Check that they are breathing—first listen by placing your ear close to their nose, and then look at their chest to see if it rises and falls. If the person is breathing normally but is not responsive, put them into the recovery position, lying on their side, unless you suspect a spinal injury. (Reasons to suspect a spinal injury include a fall or back injury, pain along the back or neck, numbness in the limbs, or lack of movement from the neck down.) The recovery position takes practice, and requires proper training to do it safely. Once you've learned, it is a great technique to practice with the whole family. If the person is not breathing, call emergency services immediately, and begin CPR.

**C** is for circulation. Make sure the person is not bleeding. Any serious bleeding needs to have pressure applied, and optimally to have the affected part raised above heart level. Watch for signs of shock— cool, clammy skin, paleness, rapid pulse and breathing, enlarged pupils, nausea, or dizziness—and seek help if you suspect shock.

## SPIRITUAL APPLICATION: *The Mysterious Placebo*

You may have heard of the "placebo effect."[19] A placebo is a medicine with no active ingredients, often used in clinical trials to assess a drug's effectiveness and side effects in people taking it compared with people who are not. The placebo effect occurs when real, measurable effects are experienced by patients despite a lack of "real" medicine. The effects can be either positive or negative—for example, a large number of patients receiving a chemotherapy placebo still lost their hair. This illustrates the potency of belief. The placebo effect has a 30% success rate on average.

Most scientists think the placebo effect is due to the body-mind connection and people's expectations. It has been shown that placebos taken by people who believe they will cure them are more effective than actual medicines taken by people who don't believe a treatment will work.

While there is still much to understand about the body-mind connection, realize that belief, hope, and trust go a long way in your healing process.

## SOUL CHALLENGE: *I Believe*

Combine the power of your beliefs with the power of your medicine. Choose a medicine you take regularly; this could be a prescription from your doctor, a flower essence, or a daily supplement.

First, spend a week keeping an informal journal about how you feel taking the medicine. Then, after a week, write on the bottle, "You heal me." *Every time you take this medicine, say this affirmation out loud. Keep an informal record of how you feel when you do this, every day for a week. How do the two weeks compare?*

## GLOBAL APOTHECARY: *Flower Essences*

The earliest written records of the use of flower essences date back to fifteenth-century alchemical texts. The sixteenth-century alchemist and healer Paracelsus said, "All medicine is in the Earth," and used the dew from flowers in his medicinal preparations. However, anecdotal and oral traditions from all over the globe, across many cultures include using flowers and plants in healing practices. The best records we have date from the Egyptian period onward. More recently, at the turn of the twentieth century, Dr. Edward Bach brought flower essences into modern consciousness.

At their core, flower essences are a vibrational medicine. They are made from imprinting the vibration of the flowers into water, and preserving it with alcohol. They have no contraindications.

Vibrational remedies work on the premise that all living cells are energy and, as such, have the potential to resonate with other energy fields. When carefully and thoughtfully prepared, each essence carries the special wisdom of its source. Flower essences share with us their plant wisdom, helping us to shift our own vibrations for health, and for spiritual growth.

See Chapter 1 for instructions on "Making a Flower Essence."

## Conjuring and Crafting

Try your hand at making a blossom essence. Different blossoms have unique medicines—for example, pears are peaceful, apples are generous, and oranges are uplifting. Choose a tree that calls to your heart. Ask Mother Nature for what you most need, and she will answer.

### SPRING BLOSSOM FLOWER ESSENCE

- Glass bowl
- Piece of cheesecloth or strainer
- Pint-size Mason jar (to store mother essence)
- 1 cup pure spring water or sacred water (water from a holy, pure source)

- Your favorite spring blossoms, alive and at the peak of their growth
- 1 cup organic vodka or brandy

Follow the "Making a Flower Essence" instructions in Chapter 1.

Take 1 drop on tongue, or 3 drops diluted in a glass of water and sipped through the day.

---

## NATURE SOUL VISION BOARD

Deepen the practice of listening to plants by creating a gorgeous sacred-inspiration pinboard for your sacred medicine space. You can use bought and found flowers, trees, and plants for this.

- Local plant guide or reference
- Journal
- Pens
- Cork or foam pinboard
- Ribbon or twine
- Pins, clothespins, or tacks
- Flowers and plants bought or collected from nature

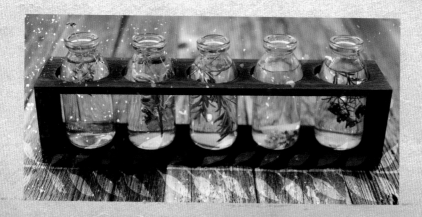

Collect a few flowers, leaves, or plants. *If wildcrafting, please follow the "Basic Rules for Honoring Nature" guidelines in the Introduction to this book.* Arrange your plant parts in posies, using the ribbon or twine. Attach them to your board.

Use your plant guide to find names and descriptions of your plants to enter in your journal. Journal about what feelings, images, colors, and memories come to you from the plants. Then you can explore the plants' meanings and uses more deeply, using repertories such as Clare Harvey's *New Encyclopedia of Flower Remedies.*

## Pairings

- Class: Pediatric first-aid class: These classes are often offered at community centers and parent outreach groups, and offer lots of great hands-on first-aid skills including CPR, recovery position, and bandaging; practiced hands-on, they will help you build confidence.

- Tool: All-terrain fabric bandages. Natural fabric, latex, and PVC-free "band-aids" are biodegradable, 100% sterile, perfect for healing little ouchies, and low-impact on Mama Earth.

- Plant Ally: Chamomile tea bags—an essential tool in any medicine cupboard, these are great for tummy aches, headaches, and can even be wetted and placed directly onto hot, tender areas of inflammation.

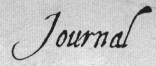

# Journal

As you begin your journey of taking the essence you made, take note of dreams, emotions, thoughts, and/or changes in your life. How does it feel when you hold the bottle? What happens when you take one drop? Where does its feeling go in your physical body? Where does it go in your emotional body? How does your spirit feel?

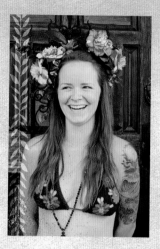

_____

_____

_____

_____

_____

_____

_____

_____

_____

_____

_____

_____

_____

_____

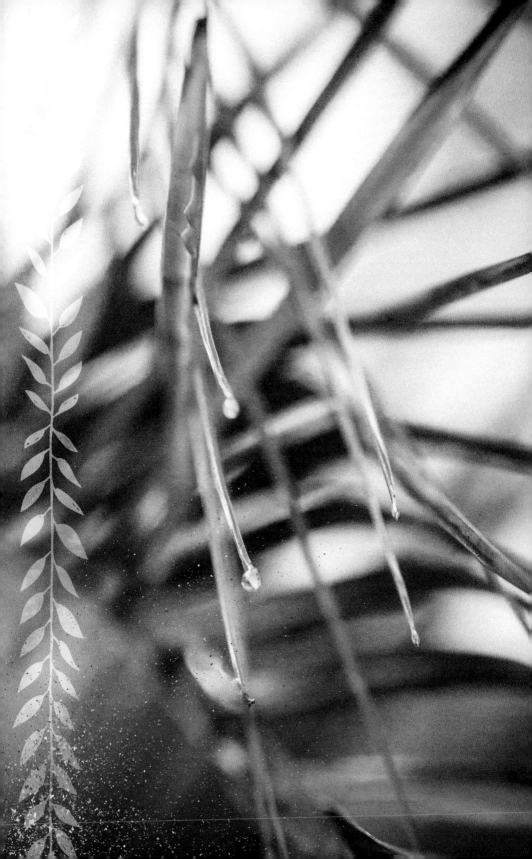

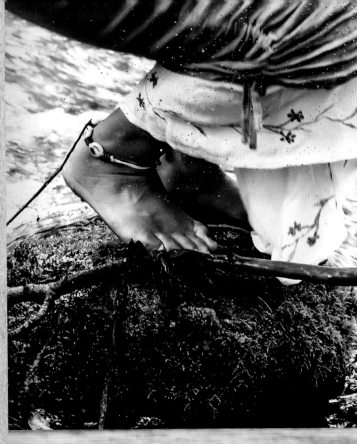

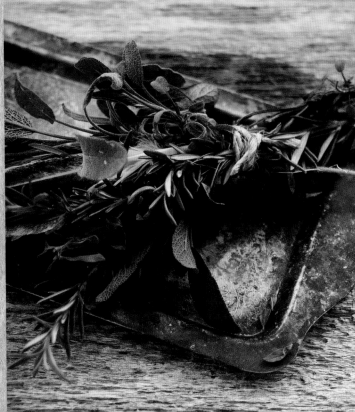

*renewal*

body of water

chapter 6

*You are a fluid being, in a constant state of motion and flow. Your cells carry information from the ancient primordial waters of the first days of this planet. In each molecule of you, there is timeless memory and knowing. This innate power helps you transmute feelings into actions, and ultimately into tangible life. You create from your eternal bubbling cauldron all that is before you. Let the tides of your soul quench your thirst for wonder and connection.*

## FAMILY WELLNESS: *Hydration*

Water is truly a magical substance. It exists in all three states of matter—liquid, solid, and gas. It is a universal solvent, and has spiritual significance across global cultures. The human body is made up of approximately 60 to 75% water, making it an intrinsic part of our being.[20]

Water is the primary medium through which nutrients and information flow through our body. It is vital in many of the body processes, including cushioning, regulating temperature, and lubricating joints and organs. It helps carry oxygen and nutrients to cells, aids digestion, dissolves many vitamins and minerals (making them bioavailable), and clears out waste products and toxins.

Physically, you take some water from foods, but the easiest way to stay hydrated is to drink water every day. Most people will get enough water from following their thirst cues if they are hydrated. If you never feel thirsty, chances are that you are dehydrated and no longer have thirst cues. Sometimes people mistake thirst for hunger, and eat when their body is really asking for water. If you are dehydrated, once you begin drinking enough water, your body needs to rebalance before it can retain the water, so it may feel like you are peeing out everything you consume! But once the cells are hydrated and able to retain the water again, you will not urinate so much.

*Dehydration signs*

- Dark and/or strong-smelling urine
- Less urine than usual

- Sunken eyes
- No tears, dry mouth, lack of saliva or sweat
- Cool, dry skin
- Fatigue
- Impaired mental functioning
- Sunken fontanel (top of head) in babies
- Listlessness or coma, in very severe cases

*How much water is enough?*

All the liquid you consume in a day contributes to your hydration. However, the purest source is always plain water. Think of it this way—if you have a plant that is thirsty, do you give it juice or tea—or do you give it pure, clean water?

Usually an average, healthy woman should drink nine eight-ounce cups of water each day, and a healthy man should drink thirteen eight-ounce cups of water a day. Some people may be taking less water due to medications or health challenges, so be sure to discuss water consumption with your care provider.

How to get more water?

- The easiest way is to carry a water bottle with you. Most people find that if they have water, they will drink it.

- Choose water as your drink at mealtimes; optimally, drink a glass of water 15–20 minutes before you eat, then only sip it throughout the meal.

- Signs that you are well hydrated include sleeping well, more energy, glowing skin, and healthy perspiration when working out.

## SPIRITUAL APPLICATION: *Water Memory*

The quality of the water in our body can change. Tears of grief, for example, are not the same as tears of joy; the chemical components and water contain different information, different memory. Emotional tears also differ from the tears used to lubricate the eye. There is evidence that water contains information and memory about emotions, and may be influenced by affirmations. Some classic experiments with this include playing different kinds of music to plants to see how they grow, or any of Dr. Emoto's experiments using positive and negative words to influence the structure of water molecules.[21]

## SOUL CHALLENGE: *Cellular Messages*

Choose two words or images and tape them onto, or put them under, two glasses of water. The words don't have to be positive and negative, just different—for example, "Courage" and "Curious," or "Happy" and "Mysterious." Leave the water overnight, and then drink the first glass the next day. Write down any changes—how you feel, your thoughts, physical sensations, etc. Then drink the second glass, and write down any changes—how you feel, your thoughts, physical sensations, etc. Compare the two.

Think about this in relation to the messages you tell yourself and how you speak to others. What communication is the water in your body receiving? What are you imprinting in the cells of others?

## GLOBAL APOTHECARY:
### *Sacred Bathing and Dew-Washing*

Sacred Bathing is taking a bath or shower prepared with the intention to cleanse body, mind, and spirit. Most medicinal traditions include some form of Sacred Bathing, as water has a long use as a spiritual cleanser. Sometimes special plants, oils, blessed waters, or salts are used. It can also be done without any special tools, as long as the intention is clear.

Dew-washing is a Celtic practice of washing your face in the spring dew. Many legends proclaim that the benefits of dew-washing include the ability to see fairies, prevent freckles and sunburn, and aid in fertility. Whatever the legendary perks, it is a refreshing and invigorating ritual to use the pure delicate moisture from the plants to wash your face and spirit. Another fun use of dew is to ask your children to collect it, and set out a fairy tea party with tiny cups of dew and fresh berries.

# *Conjuring and Crafting*

## VIBRANT FLAVORED WATERS

Yummy infused waters make drinking water more interesting, and help inspire regular consumption.

- 3-quart pitcher or water bottle
- 2½ quarts pure water
- 1–2 cups fruit or vegetables, sliced (see list below) and/or
- ¼ cup fresh herbs, roughly chopped (see list below)

*Fruit/Vegetable/Herb Ideas*—you are only limited by your imagination and palate here:

Pineapple and melon

Mango and mint

Blackberry and sage

Cucumber and strawberry

Tangerine and basil

Apple and cinnamon

Ginger and lime

Hibiscus and lemon

Citrus blossoms

Mixed herbs

Peach and nutmeg

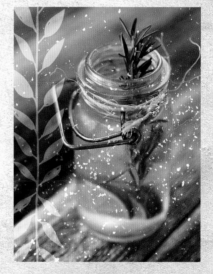

Mix ingredients in a jug, cover with pure water, and let them infuse in the fridge for 4–24 hours. Longer infusion times will result in a more potent flavor. If you tolerate cold drinks, you can serve these cold, but room temperature is fine too, and helps keep the inner fires burning.

## CLEANSING PLANT BUNDLE

Plant bundles are large bundles of herbs collected with specific intentions to make medicine for purifying. The herbs can be wildcrafted, grown in your garden, or even bought and then blessed with your prayers and intentions.

Favorites are pine, eucalyptus, rosemary, sage, thyme, fresh flowers, etc. When harvesting, tell the plants what you are making—a blessed bundle for sacred bathing—and ask them to help you cleanse what is no longer needed and to nourish you, body and soul.

- 10 or more good-size plant stalks

- Twine or hemp string

- Scissors to cut the twine

- Your prayers and intentions

Use the twine to bundle the herbs together. Bless the herbs, and ask them to help you in your cleansing. Take the bundle into the shower, and brush yourself from head to feet. Ask the water to help too. Each element will be willing to help, if approached with reverence.

When finished, offer the bundle back to the Earth with gratitude.

## Pairings

- Resource: Find A Spring, www.findaspring.org—a great website where you can find local springs that are free sources of pure water.

- Plant Ally: Citrus fruits are naturally high in electrolytes. Squeeze ¼ cup into coconut water for an excellent hydrating tonic.

- Tool: Reusable water bottles. Taking your water with you makes it easy to drink enough, and nowadays there is no need to pollute Mama Earth in the process. Invest in a decent reusable water bottle made from glass, BPA-free plastic, or aluminum-free steel, and give the landfill and oceans a break.

# Journal

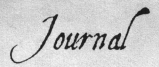

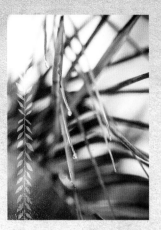

Water is an element with many faces. At times it is deep and still; at other moments it is fierce and destructive. How do your waters feel when they are in balance? How do you quench your thirst at the soul level?

_____

_____

_____

_____

_____

_____

_____

_____

_____

_____

_____

_____

_____

_____

_____

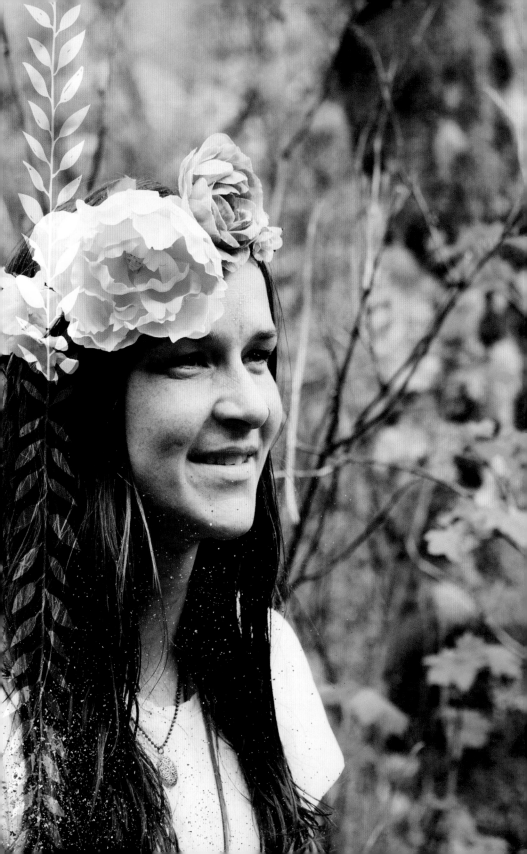

growth

*the path of transformation*

chapter 7

*Growth is a transformative energy that can literally ask everything of you. When the caterpillar encloses itself in a cocoon, it melts into a fluid state. In order to transform into a butterfly, the caterpillar comes completely undone. It breaks down into its purest essence.*

*Transformation is a similar journey. You sink into your core, dissolve your ego, and enter the place where anything is possible, where all destiny is connected. Consider carefully what Spirit asks of you in this holy place. Are you ready to wear your wings?*

## FAMILY WELLNESS: *Growing Pains*

Growing pains are pains felt in the muscles of the legs. They can be a dull ache, or a throbbing pain strong enough in some cases to wake a child up. They usually occur in children ages three to twelve, and are more common in the afternoon and evening, tending to dissipate by morning. Many studies have concluded that the cause of these pains is not rapid growth.[22] So what is the culprit? There are a few possibilities:

- **Vitamin and mineral deficiencies.** Growing is hard work, and uses up a lot of physical resources. Vitamins A, D, and B6 are all essential nutrients that support healthy bone density and muscle development. One study showed that 94% of children with growing pains were deficient in vitamin D.[23] Mineral deficiencies can be addressed with Epsom-salt baths, and increasing Bone Broth or Potassium Broth consumption (recipes in Chapter 32).

- **Poor spinal alignment** can lead to pain all over the body. As children grow, as they bump and bustle through life, the spine can get knocked out of optimal alignment. Since the skull, spine, arms, and legs are all connected, spinal adjustments can help relieve pain; chiropractic or osteopathic techniques by a trained professional experienced in working with children can be beneficial.[24]

- **Dehydration** can also be a cause of muscle pain, so if a child has been especially active, be sure they stay hydrated.

To relieve pain and soothe sore muscles, apply warmth with a hot-water bottle or Epsom-salt bath. Massage with warm oil can also be very beneficial.

## SPIRITUAL APPLICATION: *Acceptance*

Watching people you love grow and change can be challenging. Do you allow them the space and freedom to try out new ideas, new masks, new ways of being? As children become more independent, do you give them the opportunity to stretch their perceptions and live out their own soul path—which may be different from yours, and/or different from the one you think they should have?

Challenge yourself to be curious and open to how your loved ones unfold. Practicing presence—choosing to accept people exactly where they are in the moment, and not where they were yesterday or where they might be tomorrow—helps release expectations and create a spacious environment for growth.

This level of acceptance may be a lot to ask, if you don't first accept and give yourself this same open invitation for growth. Negative inner talk and self-judgment can color your personal perceptions, leading to resentment and bitterness. To attune your spirit, try the spiritual growth challenge below, and stretch into your most loving self.

## SOUL CHALLENGE: *Mirror Affirmations*

Begin by looking at yourself in the mirror. Consciously make eye contact with yourself. Folklore says that the right eye is the window to the soul, and the left eye is the window to ego, so try to focus on your right eye. Take a deep breath and smile. Look deep into your eyes and say, "I love you." *Take another deep breath and smile.*

You can build on this practice by using other simple affirmations: "You are strong." "You can do this." "I believe in you." "You are worthy."

# GLOBAL APOTHECARY: *Castor Oil*

Castor oil is made from the seeds of the castor-bean plant, *Ricinus communis*. Castor oil is a triglyceride comprised of fatty acids, 90% of which are ricinoleic acid, a unique ingredient that gives castor oil its special properties. Folk healers have found it helpful for skin issues including keratosis, dermatosis, wound healing, acne, ringworm, warts, sebaceous cysts, itching, and even hair loss. It is antibacterial, anti-inflammatory, and analgesic, and boosts lymphatic drainage.[25]

Before external application of castor oil, it is worth doing a small patch test to make sure you aren't allergic to it. It is also important to get a cold-pressed, solvent- (hexane-) free castor oil.

## *Conjuring and Crafting*

---

### CASTOR PACK FOR SORE MUSCLES

The anti-inflammatory properties of castor oil make it an excellent massage oil for relieving painful joints, nerve inflammations, and sore muscles.

- Bowl
- Hot-water bottle
- Old towels and clothes
- A comfortable, restful place to relax
- A little time and willingness to surrender
- Piece of unbleached wool or soft muslin cloth, 6–8 inches square
- Castor oil (use a good-quality, hexane-free oil)
- 3 drops of your favorite flower essence (we like pear for this)
- Non-PVC plastic wrap

Soak a piece of muslin/wool cloth in castor oil until it is totally saturated, and add a few drops of your favorite essence. While it is soaking, heat water for the hot-water bottle.

Place oil-soaked cloth over your sore joint or muscle. Then place an old washcloth or hand towel over the castor-oil cloth, to stop the oil from getting everywhere. *Castor oil stains!* Finish by wrapping the whole area in cling film to hold everything in place; this also helps keep the heat in. Add heat with a warm hot-water bottle placed over the spot. Keep this on for 45–60 minutes while you relax.

Clean the castor oil off your skin with a little baking soda and water.

You can reuse the same piece of muslin at least thirty times; just put it in the refrigerator in a plastic container and top it up each time with a little more castor oil.

## GROWTH-SPURT BATH OIL AND SALVE

First make the muscle-soothing infused bath oil below, then use the oil as the base for a salve.

### *Growth-Spurt Bath Oil*

- Pint-size bottle
- Cheesecloth or strainer
- 2 cups sweet almond or olive oil
- ¼ cup dried calendula
- ¼ cup dried lavender
- ¼ cup dried rosemary
- ¼ cup fresh ginger
- 1 lemongrass stalk
- 15 drops marjoram essential oil (only for age six and older)
- 15 drops lemongrass essential oil (only for age six and older)

Heat all the ingredients, except essential oils, in either a slow cooker or a double-boiler for 2–12 hours. Make sure the herbs don't burn; keep the heat very low and gentle.

Strain herbs out with cheesecloth, and add the essential oils. For children over the age of six, add marjoram essential oil, which is a pain reliever, and lemongrass essential oil, which is warming.

Add a few tablespoons of this oil to baths as needed.

## Growth-Spurt Salve
. . . . . . . . . . . . . . . . .

*For children age six and older only, due to essential-oil content*

- 4-ounce jar
- 2 ounces Growth-Spurt Bath Oil (above)
- 1 ounce shea butter or cocoa butter
- 1 ounce beeswax
- 25 drops peppermint essential oil
- 20 drops cajeput essential oil
- 10 drops clove essential oil

In a double-boiler, or a glass bowl set over a pan of simmering water, carefully combine beeswax, butter, and Growth-Spurt Bath Oil. Melt ingredients slowly over gentle heat. Once ingredients are completely melted, remove from heat and allow to cool a little before mixing in the other essential oils. Pour into container to finish cooling and solidifying.

Massage a small amount of salve onto sore muscles and cramps. Use as often as needed.

## "SOOTHE ME, SOAK ME" OATMEAL BATH

This bath soak is for people who are *itchy*, whether physically, mentally, or emotionally. Bergamot essential oil is a nervine, and very soothing. Calendula is a tried-and-true skin and wound healer, and lavender oil calms. The oats are known to be lubricating and anti-inflammatory, while the Epsom salts and baking soda reduce itching.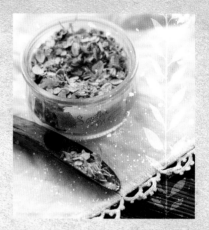

- 2½ cups fine-milled or powdered oats (or regular dry oatmeal, run through a grinder)
- 2 cups Epsom salt
- ½ cup lavender flowers
- ½ cup calendula flowers
- ¼ cup baking soda
- 25 drops bergamot essential oil
- 3 drops Spring Blossom Flower Essence (see Chapter 5)

Add essential oil and flower essence to salt, and mix well. Then add salt to the rest of the ingredients, and mix well. Store in a jar in your Sacred Medicine Cupboard.

Add a generous scoop of the soak to the bath as needed. In acute cases, such as for poison ivy, poison oak, or chickenpox, use ½ cup.

*Pairings*

- Resource: *Relax Kids* CDs. Visualization is a potent tool for coping with pain. This skill is one that can be practiced in childhood, and has lifelong benefits.

- Activity: Shiatsu—a Japanese massage therapy based in Tradition-al Chinese Medicine that helps to bring the body into balance and soothe painful muscles.

- Plant Ally: Arnica—a homeopathic remedy great for bruises and sore muscles.

# *Journal*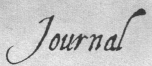

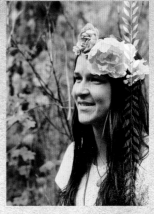

Honor the growth you experience in your
life by using this space to write a love letter
to yourself. How are you being brave and
stretching beyond your comfort zone?

_____

_____

_____

_____

_____

_____

_____

_____

_____

_____

_____

_____

_____

_____

_____

_____

_____

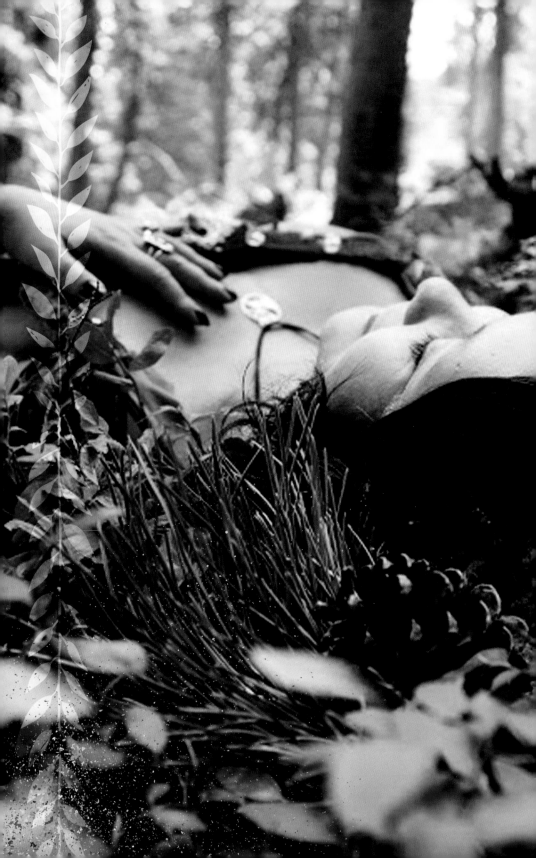

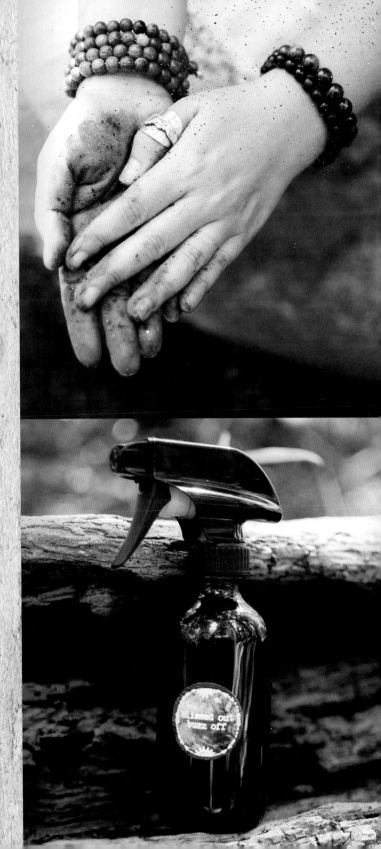

*the wild*

*what the earth sings*

chapter 8

*Once upon a time, you could talk to plants. You heard stories whispered in the rustles of leaves and the unfolding of petals. You knew in your heart what the birds sang, and where the butterfly traveled.*

*It is time to awaken this knowing. Realize once more that you are a sister to the Hawk and friend to the Willow. They have been waiting all your life for this moment. Step into the wild, and listen to the stirrings of your inner Wolf. You are part of this web, and you know it intimately.*

## FAMILY WELLNESS: *The Importance of Dirt*

In today's world, a lot of effort is spent cleaning away germs. There is an underlying fear of dirt, of the very Earth that holds you so close. Did you know that over-cleaning and sterilizing has been shown to increase rates of asthma and childhood allergies? This concept is known as the "hygiene hypothesis," and it has been well studied over the last decade.[26, 27]

It has been shown that children who don't have the opportunity to develop appropriate responses to allergens through exposure to them are more likely to experience allergies, asthma, and even auto-immune issues. This is because, in an environment that is kept too clean, their bodies never get the opportunity to develop a robust response to everyday germs and bacteria. Other studies have shown that children who grow up on farms have much lower rates of allergies and asthma. This is assumed to be because the natural microbes of their environment regularly stimulate their immune system.[28]

It is time to put down that bottle of sanitizer, and embrace the symbiotic community around us. Did you know that a certain microbe in dirt, *Mycobacterium vaccae,* triggers the release of serotonin?[29] Serotonin is an essential neurotransmitter that enhances mood and decreases anxiety. Even better, we know that the simple pleasure of interacting with earth—digging dens, baking mud pies, excavating bug palaces, even gardening—measurably elevates a child's mood and reduces their stress and worry. When in doubt, try a little outdoor play—and this goes for adults too!

## SPIRITUAL APPLICATION: *Your Wild Heart*

Each person has a wild heart. Your elemental inner being knows the language of plants and animals. But so often, the whisper of the expansive and free is ignored. It is muted by the rush of the morning school run; it is silenced with the numbing, hypnotic trance of television.

Do you pause to let the beauty of the rainbow color your soul? Are you lifted by the fragrance of the rose? Is there a part of you that is still unruly and untamed by social convention? Our wildness is the innate knowing of our Spirit and, as you know now, that wisdom is our *medicine*.

## SOUL CHALLENGE: *Your Wild Adventure*

Get in touch with your unfettered core, and that of your family. Go out in nature; put your feet and hands in the earth, and breathe deep. Explore without expectation or judgment. Ask yourself, how does your wild heart answer nature's call?

## GLOBAL APOTHECARY:
*Chaga—The Mushroom of Immortality*

Native to colder climates in the Northern Hemisphere, chaga (*Inonotus obliquus*) doesn't look very promising from the outside. It is a hard, black disc of fungus growing off the side of commonly (though not exclusively) birch trees. However, it is a potent adaptogen, and in much the same way it heals the cells in trees, it can heal us.

Chaga is immune-boosting, adaptogenic, and supportive of endocrine and nervous system balance.[30, 31, 32] It is especially nourishing to the adrenal glands. It has a long history of use in the East and in Russia; however, Western demand has put pressure on harvesting it, and there is a risk of gobbling up this precious resource if it is not used thoughtfully. Ground chaga powder is both economical and environmentally friendly, as it generates much less waste. Always seek ethical sources.

---

## BUG BITE 101

Bugs have been biting people since the relationship started! It is kinda part of being in nature. There are some pretty scary diseases spread by things like mosquitoes and ticks, so it is good to have some ideas of prevention and care. Here is a list of basic bug-kit items, plus notes on how to use them.

*What you need for your bug kit*

· · · · · · · · · · · · · · · · · · · · · · · ·

- Spray bottle
- Small lip-balm-size container (for your charcoal paste)
- Activated charcoal capsules
- Spring water
- Plastic credit card or similar card
- Cloth to make compresses or wrap ice
- Vinegar
- Baking soda
- Manuka honey
- Grapefruit-seed extract or tea tree oil
- Your favorite essential oils—check out the list below, and make sure they are age-appropriate if you have children.
- An oil or solvent (such as vodka or witch hazel) to dilute your essential oils

### Activated charcoal paste

Black paste helps pull out the toxins that cause inflammation, swelling, and itching. Mix the powder from 2–3 capsules of charcoal with enough water to make a paste (usually about 1 teaspoon). Spread thickly over the bite. Wipe with a wet cloth after about 30 minutes.

### Ice

Ice, or a very cold compress, soothes the itch, reduces inflammation and swelling, and eases the pain of bites and stings. Place lightly crushed ice into the cloth, or wet the cloth with very cold water, and apply to the bite. A bag of frozen veggies works for this too!

### Credit card

Carefully and gently remove bee stingers by scraping along the surface of the skin with a credit card. Don't reach for the tweezers or tongs—grabbing and squeezing the stinger causes more venom to be pumped into the wound. If the area is inflamed after removal, activated charcoal paste or a topical antiseptic like manuka honey or grapefruit-seed extract may help. While there is no scientific evidence to back it up, in many places vinegar is used to neutralize wasp stings, and a baking-soda paste is used to neutralize bee stings.

### Fresh basil

Though you can't keep fresh leaves in a bug-bite kit, rubbing a fresh basil leaf on a mosquito bite or insect sting helps reduce inflammation and soothe pain. Mozzies don't like the smell of basil either!

## Spider bites

As long as it isn't a poisonous spider bite, simply clean the bite well and apply a good antimicrobial, antibacterial treatment such as tea tree oil, grapefruit-seed extract, or manuka honey. Keep an eye on it for signs of infection—redness, swelling, a ring around the bite mark, or excessive pain. These are signs that it is time to get it checked by your doctor. Trust your instincts.

## Tick bites

Ticks are avoided by wearing long sleeves and pants when out in nature. Early detection and removal of biting ticks within twenty-four hours has been shown to reduce risk of Lyme disease, so it is good to check right after getting home. They like warm, moist spots, so check the groin, armpits, hairline, and all around the torso.

*To remove a tick:* Use tick-removal tweezers, some of which even come with a magnifying glass. Always remove the entire tick, including the head, which burrows beneath the skin surface. Do this by taking hold of the body with the tweezers and pulling out in one steady, gentle lift. If you are in an area with Lyme disease, you can save the tick by placing it in a bag in the freezer so it can be tested.

## Essential oils to repel bugs

**Mosquitos:** Peppermint, lemongrass, *Eucalyptus globulus,* rosemary, lavender, rose geranium (Pelargonium), citronella, clove, bergamot

**Ticks:** Tansy, rose geranium (specifically *Pelargonium capitatum x radens),* eucalyptus, sweet myrrh

**Gnats:** Rose geranium, peppermint, citronella, *Eucalyptus globulus*

## BLISSED-OUT BUZZ OFF! MISTER

This "do-it-yourself" bug repellent, with no yucky endocrine-disrupting chemicals,[33] is our favorite blend for children.

- Lavender essential oil

- Rose geranium (Pelargonium) essential oil

- Citronella essential oil

- Clove essential oil (age three and up) or eucalyptus essential oil (age ten and up)

For children over the age of three, you can add clove. For children over the age of ten, you can add eucalyptus—but only add one of these, for a total of four essential oils.

Mix 5 drops of each oil (for a sensitive-skin dilution) or 10 drops of each oil (for a strong dilution) into 2 teaspoons of vodka or witch hazel, and mix into ¼ cup fresh spring water. Place in misting bottle, and spritz exposed skin when outdoors. Apply liberally every 2–3 hours in areas with a high concentration of bugs.

## CHAGA CHAI

*This chai recipe, shared with us by our favorite wild-hearted wise woman, Nikiah Seeds at the Red Moon Mystery School, is a family tradition from her mother-in-law.*

### Chaga Chai Powder

- ¼ cup cinnamon pieces

- ⅛ cup cloves

- ¼ cup black peppercorns

- ¼ cup green cardamom

- 4–6 dried anise flowers

- 1 Tablespoon nutmeg, grated

- ¾ cup dried ginger powder
- ¼ cup chaga powder

Dry-roast all ingredients *except* the nutmeg, ginger, and chaga in a pan (preferably cast-iron) on low heat for about 5 minutes, until you can smell the spices heating up and releasing their oils. Remove them to a plate and allow them to cool.

Once they are cool to the touch, grind them into very fine 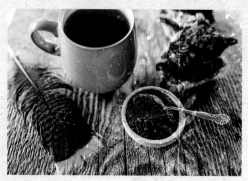 powder in a coffee or spice grinder. Then add the grated nutmeg, ginger, and chaga. Mix well and store in an airtight jar. Now you can make a perfect cup of chai tea anytime!

### Chaga Chai Tea

* * * * * * * * * * * *

*Makes 4 cups*
- 1–2 cups milk, any kind—dairy, soy, almond, etc.
- ¼ cup Chaga Chai Powder (above)
- 2–3 crushed cardamom pods
- 1–2 small cinnamon sticks
- 3–4 black peppercorns
- 3–4 cloves
- 1–3 slices fresh ginger, depending on how spicy you like it
- 2–3 Tablespoons of sugar—or more!
- 4 Indian black tea bags such as Assam

In a large pot, mix 3 cups of water with one cup of milk. (If you like a milkier chai, try 2 cups each of water and milk.)

Add ¼ cup of the Chaga Chai Powder that you just made (above), plus the additional spices to make it even spicier, and the sugar. This is the traditional way. My mother-in-love, Azra, swears by adding this amount of sugar, if not more, and it is surprising how it mixes into the chai after it has boiled, making it almost caramelized. You can replace the sugar with coconut sugar, and it is also okay to omit it altogether if you are avoiding sugar.

Let the mixture come to a boil; then turn down the burner, and bring it back up again, for a total of 3 times.

Now you may add your tea bags—4 total, and let it steep several minutes before straining and serving. We like to use India tea, as it makes a good strong pot. It is said that giving your guests of honor a cardamom pod or anise pod added to their chai is a gesture of respect, and I believe it, as both of my in-laws/in-loves like to chew on the pods and enjoy them very much. And they are always guests of honor in our house!

## Pairings

- Resource: Your local botanical garden. Get to know your neighborhood plants and critters by visiting those cultivating them.
- Book: *Women Who Run with the Wolves* by Clarissa Pinkola Estes—a classic call to the wild for the modern woman.
- Music: "Mother Protect," by Niki and the Dove—dance with your wild heart and allow this song to awaken your inner Eagle.

# *Journal*

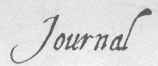

Nature is experiential; you connect with all your senses. Go outside and observe something in nature through the lens of each sense—your eyes, your ears, your hands, your nose, your heart, and your intuition. How was each one different? What did you learn?

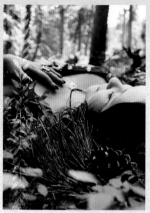

_____

_____

_____

_____

_____

_____

_____

_____

_____

_____

_____

_____

_____

_____

_____

_____

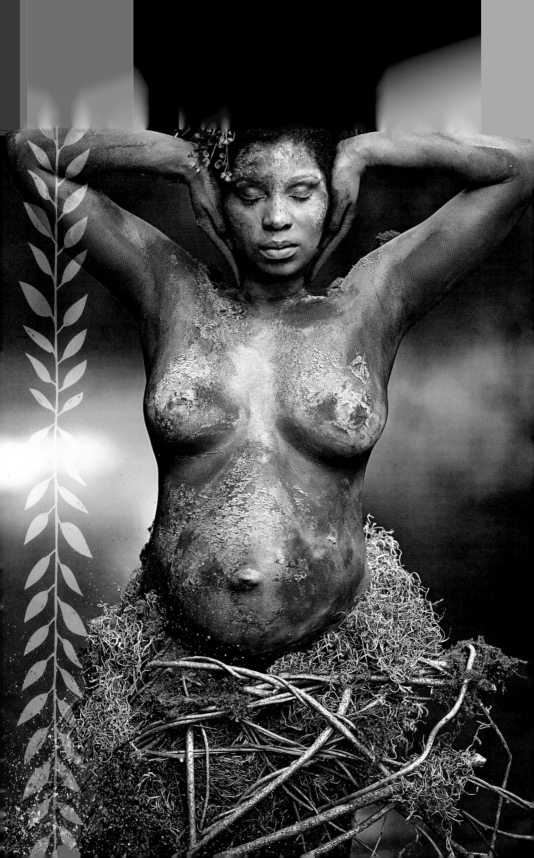

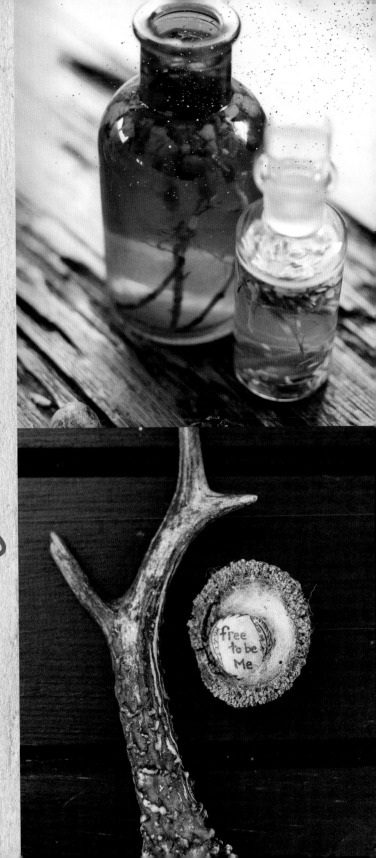

# magic

## weaving the roots

chapter 9

*Sometimes you get to pull back the curtain and spy the inner workings of this mysterious universe. Things like unexplained intuition, déjà vu, or astounding synchronicities just cannot be denied. It seems at times that the more you understand, the less you know. The vastness of what we still do not understand about the universe is immense, and within the inner workings of the cosmos lie answers to questions we do not even know to ask. You are a great soul in this mysterious dance, and are connected to the enormous web of life, a part of the source of all existence.*

*This truth exists even when you forget, even when it is hidden, even when you did not know it was there. This is our call to you to remember that you are an essential part of this weaving. This connection is the foundation of all magic. We are throwing down the universal-question gauntlet—do you believe in magic? Really believe? Are you open to the knowing (and unknowing) of the universal mysteries that abound?*

## FAMILY WELLNESS: *Life-Force*

Over fifty different cultures from all around the world have been identified as having a concept of "life-force" or "life-energy" in some form. Specifically, these include *ki* (Japanese), *chi* or *qi* (Chinese), *neyatoneyah* (Lakota Sioux), *ruach* or *roohah* (Hebrew), *rooh* (Persian), and *lung* (Tibetan). We already met *prana* (Sanskrit) in the early pages of this book.

Life-force is a vital energy that awakens your consciousness and inhabits every molecule of your being. It flows through every part of you, and connects you to the greater network of the universe. In Chinese Medicine it is said, *"The energy flows where the mind goes."* This means that if you want something to change, you send your mind or thoughts on a mission to make it happen, and the energy, or *qi*, will follow. If you can imagine it, then it can happen.

This understanding of how energy moves is the same in many therapeutic practices, and has been explored by science. Quantum theory describes how the observer influences the thing observed.[34]

This could mean that the very act of observing (sending your mind on a stated quest) may influence the world around you—wow! Science has also shown that you are not just made up of Newtonian matter. You are living cells, which are made up of movement, connection, and vibration.[35]

With your spiritual connection to the universe, your physical self has the potential to influence the whole environmental system, the whole web around you, which includes pretty much everything—thoughts, feelings, food, spiritual practices, exercise, nature, and relationships.

Your ability to influence energetics does not mean you have superpowers to control everything that happens to you. You don't. There are way too many variables to account for. Scary, hard, intense things can happen at anytime without your conscious approval. Loved ones get sick, accidents happen, global unrest ensues, and the list goes on.

What you absolutely do have control over is your response to these things. And it is your reaction to the tough stuff that unveils the true magic that lies within your reach, which is your personal brand of medicine.

## Spiritual Application: *Magic*

Magic is an attempt to understand, experience, and influence the world using rituals, symbols, actions, gestures, and language. Magic can include storytelling, imagination, intention, touch, and ritual. In pagan traditions, a spell is literally linking letters together to make words that spell out your intentions; this pure prose expresses and shapes your understanding and experience of the world. This perception, in turn, influences the outcome of your experience. And that is magic—right?

What are you doing when you pray? You are sending words up to your god/goddess for help or assistance. Praying is something of a lost art in our busy world, but it is a sacred and important one. When we pray, we are in communication with Spirit. We are sending our thoughts and therefore our intention out (or *in*, as the case may be) to connect with Source—the energy of all life, which is pure, divine, abundant, and life-affirming.

## SOUL CHALLENGE: *Wands*

Are you ready to believe? There are few things more readily identifiable with magic than a wand. A wand is simply a piece of wood that fits in your hand and is the right length for you. For most general purposes, there are no real rules about what type of wood to use, or how long it should be—all you have to do is trust Mother Earth to call you to the right stick.

Start by going outside. Wait for your significant stick to make itself known. Choose your stick wisely, as this wand is what you will use to connect with your magic and aid the flow of your energy during a ritual or prayer. The process of crafting a wand is really straightforward—it can be as easy as finding a stick outside and deciding it's finished, leaving it raw and untouched.

You can also choose to adorn it with string, beads, feathers, or copper spirals. You can carve it, if you feel called to that. You may find a stone or a crystal to adorn the end of your wand, and this may magnify the energy, helping to direct your intention more clearly. You can also peel the bark off the wand and polish it lovingly with a layer of beeswax and essential oils.

Once you have your wand ready, hold it tightly and focus all of your intention on your goal. If your hands get hot, cold, or tingly, this is a sign that energy is moving. When you have your goal crystalclear in your mind's eye, ask for the wand's help in making it so.

Point the wand to the sky and say this invocation: *As it harm none, my will be done. May the ancestors in the sky aid me.*

Point your wand to the Earth and say: *As above, so below; may the guardians of the Earth honor my vision.*

Point the wand at your heart and say: *As my heart is open and right action flows, so does my work.*

Finally, point the wand away from you and say: *As I will it, so shall it be to the greatest good of all concerned. As I will it, so shall it be. As I will it, so shall it be.*

## GLOBAL APOTHECARY: *Root Chakra*

The root chakra, called *muladhara,* sits at the base of the pelvic floor and extends up into the lower three vertebrae of the spine. The name can be translated as "root base." The root chakra is really focused on basic needs such as your right to exist, to be loved, and to be embodied. It is a chakra that deals with stability, balance, and grounding. The sound *"lam"* and the color red help to open and bring balance to this anchoring chakra.[36]

## *Conjuring and Crafting*

It's time to create some everyday magic with these vibration-raising goodies.

---

## CRYSTAL CARE: GROUNDING, BALANCING, AND PROGRAMMING BASICS

We recommend and use crystals regularly. Crystals are wonderful at supporting you in your deep work; all you really need to do is request specific help from a crystal that resonates with whatever energies you are working with.

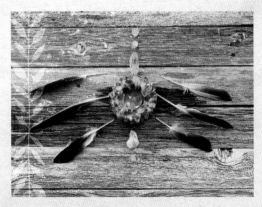

When you find a crystal that resonates with your intention, you can ask it to help you in some specific way. This kind of crystal task-assignment is called "programming," much as the silicon crystals in computers get programmed. Here are some top tips for working with these guides.

### *Basic crystal cleaning and programming instructions*

1. **Clean your crystal.** Cleaning is not for washing away negative energy; it is for helping your crystals to return to their own natural, harmonious vibration. You can help your crystals retune to this natural vibration by leaving them in the sunlight, or placing them in a bowl of salt, or burying them in the earth. Not all crystals should be washed in water, either; a good rule of thumb is never to wash any crystal whose name ends in "-ite," as these tend to be porous and can be damaged by water.

2. **Sit with your crystal in a quiet place.** Hold your crystal in your hand, and bring it up to your heart. Close your eyes and, with an exhalation, say your intention to your crystal.

3. **Hold your crystal until you feel a connection.** This relationship can be perceived through warmth, images, or feelings—it is different for everyone.

4. **Maintain the connection.** Carry your crystal with you, and every time you touch it you will be reminded of your path.

---

## ROOTED ESSENCE

Try your hand at making an essence to support your connection to the Earth's life-force. Choose a tree, plant, or crystal that calls to your heart. Ask Mother Nature for what you need most, and she will answer.

- Glass bowl
- Piece of cheesecloth or strainer

- Pint-size Mason jar (to store mother essence)
- 1 cup pure spring water or sacred water, water from a Holy, Pure Source
- Nature item to support your grounding work; if a plant, choose one that is alive and at the peak of its growth
- 1 cup organic vodka or brandy

Follow the "Making a Flower Essence" instructions in Chapter 1. Take 1 drop on the tongue, or 3 drops diluted in a glass of water and sipped through the day.

## Pairings

- Book: *How to See Faeries* by John Matthews, illustrated by Brian Froud—a magical and mischievous guide to the fair folk.
- Resource: Mountain Rose Herbs—an ethical and wise place to buy herbs online.
- Crystal: Emerald—a heart stone that inspires magic, creativity, and psychic awareness, and helps connect with astral realms.

# Journal

Do you believe in magic? What does
magic mean to you?

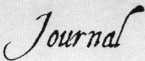

_____

_____

_____

_____

_____

_____

_____

_____

_____

_____

_____

_____

_____

_____

_____

_____

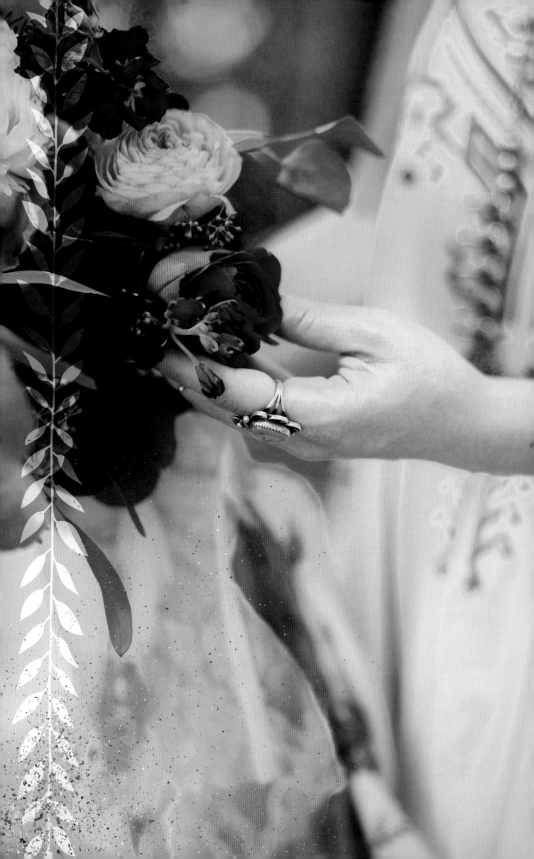

# PART TWO

# Summer

Sun-kissed and radiant, you dance to the sway of the heat,

Feet pounding, heart beating, eyes glistening.

The rising pulse of the season lifts you on a natural high.

Summer comes resplendent and alluring,

To set your wings on fire and ignite the

Passions of your soul.

Welcome the flames, the intoxicating lure

Of a life lived fully.

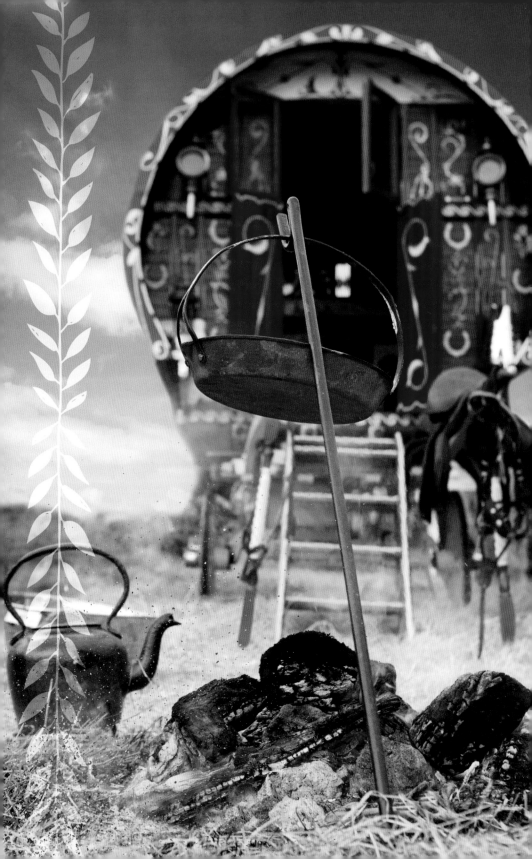

# midday

*illuminating all of our senses*

chapter 10

*Allow the golden liquid warmth of the midday sun to caress your bare skin. Tingle with the sensation of your inner fires glowing, heat licking upwards from your core. You are a luminous being, full of passion and vitality. You burn with inspiration and excitement. Here in the full light of day, you use all of your senses to tune in and fully experience this voluptuous moment. Inhale it! Taste it! See it! Know It! Expose your divinity and sparkle—it is time to shine!*

## FAMILY WELLNESS: *What are the Five Senses?*

- **Touch** is the dance between your skin, your environment, and your neurotransmitters. This sensation is about exploration, discovery, and experience.

- **Sight** is the eyes and brain translating the myriad of imagery, pictures, dreams, and visions into cohesive meaning. This sense is about color and expression.

- **Hearing** is the auditory absorption of information. It is about listening and communication.

- **Taste** is the bridge between your internal "gut" wisdom and your outer world. Often, taste is a subtle statement of your underlying health.

- **Smell** is the time-traveler of the senses. It can take you right back to a sweet memory or a forgotten fear with one quick whiff.[37]

If you lose a sense, the other senses will take up its role. You can hone or diminish your senses as needed. Parents of children with increased sensitivity know it is important to limit the amount of sensory stimuli. It is worth considering that picky eaters may just have "super-palates," and that what they eat simply does not taste the same to them as it does to you. Children who react strongly and emotionally to loud noises may be hearing something different. Not all children can cope with the fast-moving pictures of television, or with a sudden touch, because the sensation is just too strong. Senses are a gift unique to each person, and deserve to be honored as such.

## SPIRITUAL APPLICATION: *The Sixth Sense*

There is another sense. It has many names—the sixth sense, intuition, inner knowing. It is when your very cells comprehend your purpose, and vibrate with certainty. It is when you feel truth in your bones, your gut, and your heart. It is information you download without conscious reasoning. It is your link to the Divine Mind, open and shining through your awareness. As previously stated, Divine Mind is the place in you that holds trust and love. When you access your Divine Mind, anything becomes possible, and you have all the information you need.

## SOUL CHALLENGE: *Mindful Senses*

Develop your sixth sense, and hone your other senses through mindfulness practice. Sit comfortably and close your eyes. Notice your breathing; how does your breathing feel today? Notice the sounds and sensations around you; take in any smells, or the feeling of sun on your skin. As you settle into your awareness, notice your thoughts and feelings. Are you able to observe your internal landscape with openness? By paying attention to all the ways you receive information, you encourage your intuition to communicate with you.

## GLOBAL APOTHECARY: *Healing Touch*

Touch is a healing. **Sometimes it is all that is needed.**

Have you ever bumped your knee, and put your hands there to touch the pain? Has a child been hurt, and you held them while they cried? These are both common forms of "healing touch." Healing touch is the laying-on of hands, or using physical contact if you don't have hands to relieve pain, whether physical, emotional, or spiritual. It is your birthright as a conscious being on this planet; all people have this skill to varying degrees. All it takes to use this tool is a little practice and clear intention. Some good practices to keep in mind are to ask permission before you touch, be gentle, and always touch with the intention of the highest good for all involved.

# *Conjuring and Crafting*

Avocado is a superfood. It is full of phytonutrients including oleic acid, lutein, folic acid, vitamins A, E, K, B6, and C, and monounsaturated fats and glutathione. An avocado also has twice the potassium of a banana. It's time to play with your senses, feeding yourself inside and out.

## AVOCADO TOAST

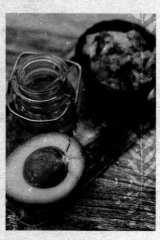

Play with your senses of taste and smell.

- I ripe avocado
- I piece of bread (I like organic sprouted sourdough)
- I Tablespoon pomegranate seeds
- I Tablespoon crushed nuts such as almonds or pistachios
- Pink Himalayan salt, to taste
- Black pepper, to taste

Toast the bread. Cut the avocado in half, and spread it on the toast. Sprinkle with pomegranate seeds and nuts. Season with salt and pepper to taste.

Eat for breakfast, lunch, or dinner, savoring the taste and the sensations of texture.

## AVOCADO FACE MASK

Play with your senses of touch and sight.

- 4-ounce jar with lid
- 2 avocados
- ¼ cup raw, local honey

- 3 drops white lotus or iris flower essence

Mash the avocado well, and mix in the honey. Add 3 drops of your flower essence, and mix again.

Use by applying gently to your face—it is wonderful to rub right into your skin. Leave it on for 10 minutes or so, and then rinse well with fresh water.

---

## SERENITY AURIC MISTER FOR SENSITIVE PEOPLE

Today's world is overloaded with sensory input, and it is easy to get overwhelmed physically, mentally, and energetically. Here is a recipe for an auric mister to calm the senses.

- 1-ounce mister bottle
- 3 drops flower essence—choose one of these: yarrow, silver, kunzite, Rescue Remedy or Homemade "To-the-Rescue" Flower Essence (see Chapter 28), angelsword, pear
- 5–10 drops total of your favorite supportive essential oils—choose one or two: chamomile, clary sage, lavender, frankincense, sandalwood
- 1 teaspoon solvent (vodka, witch hazel, or vanilla extract)
- 1 ounce pure spring water
- Small tumble-stone turquoise crystal

Use 5 drops of essential oil for a sensitive dilution, or 10 drops for a standard dilution. Mix oils, flower essences, and solvent together. Add water and crystal. Leave on your altar to charge the mixture.

When it feels ready to you, put liquid in misting bottle, and mist around your space and your aura as needed.

*Pairings*

- Skill: Reiki attunements are a great way to build confidence with your healing touch.

- Medicine Cupboard Staple: Weleda Rose Oil delights all the senses. Roses have one of the highest vibrations in nature, and stimulate awareness and consciousness.

- Flower Essence: Goddess Awakens essence by Soul Tree Essences— this quince essence activates the divine chalice within us, tapping into our sensual creativity.

# Journal

Choose something beautiful, such as a flower, or fifteen minutes with your child, and experience the moment with all of your senses. Which senses do you use most? Did you receive any information from your Divine Mind?

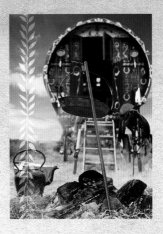

_____
_____
_____
_____
_____
_____
_____
_____
_____
_____
_____
_____
_____
_____
_____
_____
_____
_____
_____
_____

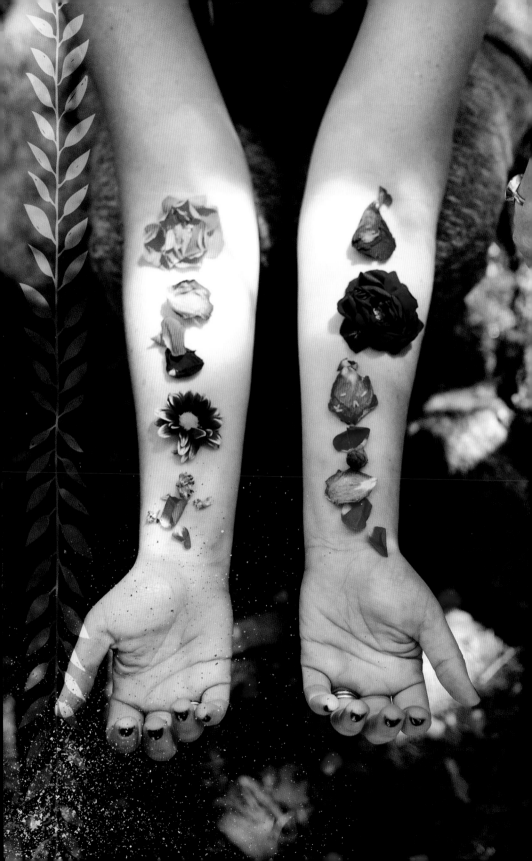

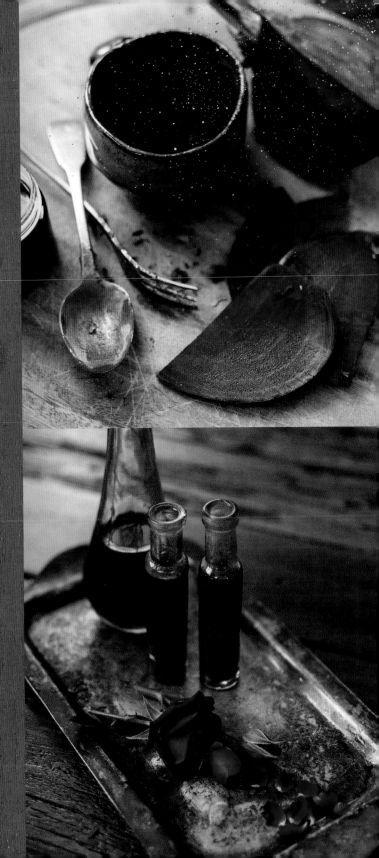

# tantra

*the ooh & aah*

## chapter II

*The energy of the summer sun brings forth your will and passions, and begs you to dive into the heat of your desires. Sinking into the drippingly delicious place of pleasure, you seek to understand what moves you, and how experiencing the tingle of ecstasy can bring you to an ecstatic spiritual experience.*

*Make no mistake about it—pleasure is a powerful force; it can drive you to places unknown that can either serve your highest good or act to its detriment if out of balance. Allowing yourself the space to breathe in sensuality and deeply drink tantric moments can awaken parts of you that you did not even know were dormant. Being turned on by your life is healthy for the soul. It is sacred medicine that feeds the core of who you are.*

## FAMILY WELLNESS: *Pleasure is Medicine*

Pleasure, whether physical, emotional, or spiritual, is a medicine that washes over all layers of your being. When you experience pleasure, your brain is flooded with feel-good neurotransmitters such as serotonin and dopamine.[38, 39] The uplift from pleasure also stimulates endorphins, which are natural painkillers in the body, and oxytocin, which is the love hormone of connection and bonding. Pleasure is one of the fires of creation, and it can make you feel alive and awake in every way. This vitality spills out into your daily life and work.

## SPIRITUAL APPLICATION: *Receiving*

Often the flow of pleasure is out of balance in people's lives. Many people tend to feel more comfortable giving rather than receiving. In terms of pleasure, how good are you at receiving? Are you able to fully embody your pleasure without guilt or shame? Let's think about three areas where you could receive pleasure, and how well you are doing in these. Be kind to yourself—but if there is room to receive more, allow yourself the opportunity.

- **Compliments.** When someone throws an emotional rose at your feet, say thank you, breathe, and let in the pleasure of being seen for your light and talents.

- **Self-care.** If there were no limits, what would you give yourself? Explore luscious ways to meet your pleasure needs. How often do you say YES to that new dress, or getting a massage in the middle of the week just because you want one?

- **Sexy time.** Do you allow yourself to receive pleasure, and do you feel comfortable asking your partner for what you want? What would your sexual life look like with more play pleasure infused into the routine? Go on! You deserve it!

## SOUL CHALLENGE: *Saying Yes to Pleasure*

We all have sexual energy that courses through our bodies and needs to be expressed. But some of us hold sexuality scars that are hard to heal, and others may be fearful of allowing ourselves to truly feel deep pleasure in moments of true surrender. Ask yourself, what is pleasure like for you? Do you take it on and say YES, or do you hide from it, feeling embarrassed by your needs?

In an attempt to open up this place of pleasure within, sit in meditation using the Lotus Mudra to help stimulate opening pleasure within: The bases of your hands are together, with your pinkies and thumbs touching, while all other fingers are open like the petals of a flower. Repeat the mantra *"Om mani padme hum,"* which invokes the "jewel in the lotus."

Next, try writing a sexy, sexy poem for your beloved, and read it during pleasure playtime.

## GLOBAL APOTHECARY: *Sacral Chakra*

*Svadhishthana,* the sacral chakra, means "home to the self." It is located below the belly button and above the pubic bone. It contains the sexual organs and lower intestinal tract. It is the sacred cauldron of creation, and home to our sense of abundance, pleasure, and joy. The sound *"vam"* and the color orange help to open and balance this powerhouse of a chakra.[40]

### Yab-yum posture

Try sitting in the *yab-yum* tantric pose with your beloved. Yab-yum (which means "mother/father") is the union between wisdom (feminine) and compassion (masculine); it is the coming together of the sacral energies. Try this tantric pose, and see how it feels.

Have your beloved sit in cross-legged position, and then sit on top of his legs with your legs wrapped around his or her body. Place your foreheads together, opening your third-eye chakras and allowing your hands to move about the other's body. Do not kiss or indulge in any further sexual play—only touch, and breathe each other's breath. Let the tantric energy flow pulsate between you and get your kundalini rising. This is an amazing lovers' practice that you can use as a precursor to your love-making pleasure journey.

## Conjuring and Crafting

### LOVE POTION

*This recipe is a gift from Sarah Josey
of Golden Poppy Herbal Apothecary.*

The herbs in this potion have long been considered aphrodisiacs. They include some herbs that are relaxing, some that are stimulating, and some that increase blood circulation—all of which are necessary for a romantic evening.

- Large Mason jar
- Cheesecloth
- Storage bottle
- Large pot
- ¼ ounce kava-kava root
- ¼ ounce ashwagandha root

- ¼ ounce passionflower leaf
- ¼ ounce damiana leaf
- ¹⁄₁₀ ounce rose petals
- ¹⁄₁₀ ounce cardamom pods
- ¹⁄₁₀ ounce cinnamon bark chips
- ¹⁄₁₀ ounce whole cloves
- ¹⁄₁₀ ounce dry ginger root
- ¹⁄₁₀ ounce star anise
- Brandy (about 10 ounces)
- Honey to sweeten

Place all the herbs in a large Mason jar, and shake well to mix. Pour enough brandy over the herbs to cover them, and then add an additional inch of brandy above the herbs. After the first few days you may need to add more brandy, as the herbs soak some of it up, which is perfectly fine.

Seal and label the jar, and place it out of the sun. Shake it daily for two weeks, each time thinking of nothing but self-love and nurturing. At the end of the two weeks, strain the brandy out through cheesecloth. Squeeze out as much as possible, and reserve the liquid for later.

Place the herbs into a large pot and just cover them with water (about 14 ounces). Simmer with the lid on until the water is reduced by half. Strain out the herbs through the cheesecloth, squeezing out as much liquid as possible. Compost the herbs. Add the infused brandy to the warm herbal tea, and stir in honey to your liking. Place in a jar and label.

Pull this out to share on sexy and loving occasions. As a sipping cordial, pour 1–2 ounces into a pretty cup of your choice, top with pomegranate juice, and sip while thinking loving thoughts. It can also be mixed with champagne for an interesting cocktail.

## SELF-LOVE ELIXIR

Take this elixir once a day over the next month to raise your vibration and support your beautiful unfolding into pleasure.

- ¼ cup organic wild roses, dried
- 1 Tablespoon dried jasmine flowers
- 1 cinnamon stick
- Zest of 1 orange
- ½ cup raw cacao nibs
- 2 cups raw honey from beloved bees

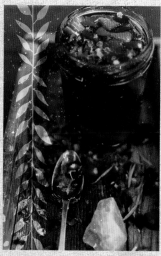

Pour your honey into a double-boiler, or in a heatproof bowl over a pot of gentling simmering water. Keep the heat low, to gently warm your honey. Then add all other ingredients.

Turn off the heat and cover. Let your honey sit for 1–6 hours—the longer it sits, the stronger it will be. Taste it to see when it is ready; when it tastes amazing, you are good to go! Strain the flowers and spices from the honey. Use a fine-mesh strainer over a large bowl, or strain directly into jars.

Take a spoonful every day to remind you of sweet pleasure.

## BEET-SYRUP LIP TINT

An edible lip tint with a hint of mystery.

- 4-ounce container
- 1½ Tablespoons beeswax pastilles
- 3 Tablespoons cocoa butter

- 1 Tablespoon coconut oil
- 4 ounces beet juice
- 3 drops of juicy flower essences such as pomegranate, queen orchid, or The Goddess Awakens
- ¼ teaspoon rose extract

Cook down the beet juice until reduced to about half.

Pour everything except the flower essences into a double-boiler, or in a heatproof bowl over a pot of gently simmering water. Keep the heat low, to gently melt everything together. Once melted, turn off heat and add the flower essences.

Pour into jar and allow to cool completely.

Apply to your lips with soft fingertips.

## Pairings

- Book: *Urban Tantra: Sacred Sex for the Twenty-First Century* by Barbara Carrellas
- Crystal: Shiva lingam—this crystal helps to bring balance to the union of masculine and feminine divine energies. It also helps awaken kundalini energy.
- Music: "Swoon" by Rising Appalachia—a super-sexy-sexy song to bring into your love-making time.

# Journal

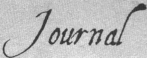

Use this space to explore your pleasures and
your ability to receive.

_____

_____

_____

_____

_____

_____

_____

_____

_____

_____

_____

_____

_____

_____

_____

_____

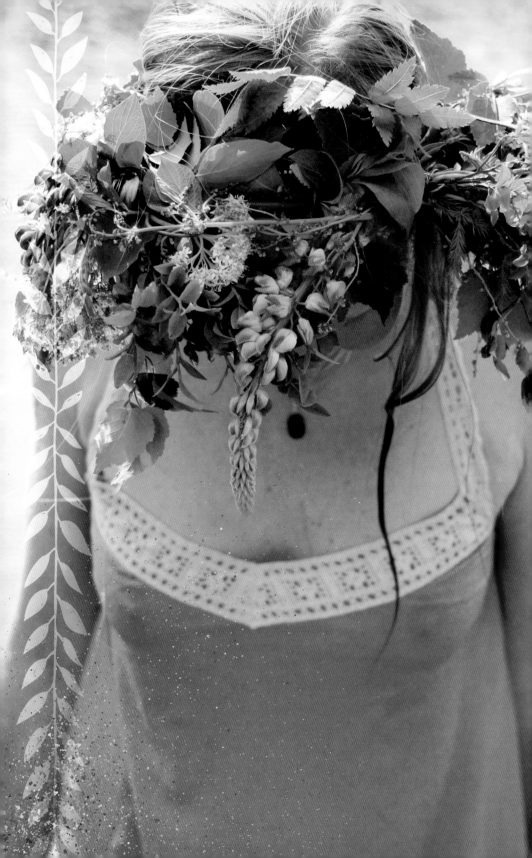

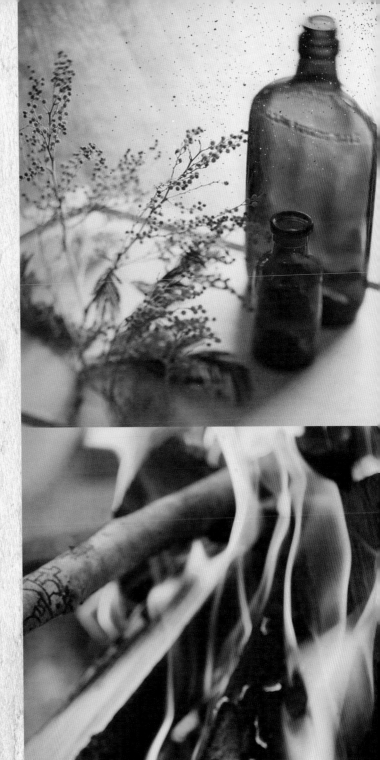

*summer solstice*

*luscious celebrant*

**chapter 12**

*This moment is the cresting peak of the year. Everything around you is alive and humming in the throes of summer passion. You feel lush, uncensored, and bold. Drink deep and long of every ounce of this celestial elixir. You are the luscious celebrant, the reigning queen of the season, full of energy, light, and golden inspiration. Open your sensuality and expansive heart space to experience the fires of the Summer Solstice.*

## FAMILY WELLNESS: *Heart Health*

The heart is divided into two pumps. The right pump pushes blood returning from the organs and tissues into the lungs. The lungs oxygenate the blood and remove carbon dioxide waste. Then the left pump pulls the fresh blood from the lungs and into the body again. The heart beats without conscious intention; it serves us all day and night from soon after our conception to our last moment in our bodies. In some medicine traditions, the heart is so important that it is considered the seat of the soul. A healthy heart allows you to connect your inner world to your outer world with quiet confidence.

### *Heart-healthy tips*[41]

- **The heart is a muscle, and it gets stronger when you use it.** Exercise is a great way to do this—swimming, running, walking, or team sports are all excellent ways to feel good and get your heart moving.
- **Feed your heart with care and love.** The heart does not do well with processed foods and sugar, or trans fats. Trans fats are artificial, processed fats usually used in packaged food to help extend shelf life. Avoid these if possible!
- **Calm and soothe your whole body.** Much research has shown that inflammation is a major trigger for cholesterol to line the arteries. Any inflammation in the body is a sign that, in general, things are out of balance. Inflammation can be reduced through eating lots of fresh fruits and vegetables, and making healthy lifestyle choices in general.

- **Stay hydrated.** Hydration affects your blood pressure and how hard your heart has to work. Keeping yourself refreshed with water keeps your organs working optimally. It is no coincidence that nature provides an abundance of watery fruits to eat this time of year, so dive in.
- **Slow down and breathe.** Your heart is affected by stress and strong emotions. Balance stressors with a pause if you can. Take a deep breath, give yourself or a loved one a hug, and know that if need- ed, it is okay to create some emotional space if needed for the over- all health of your heart.

## SPIRITUAL APPLICATION: *Elevate the Mundane*

Summer Solstice is the longest day of the year. Traditionally, Celts honored this season as a time of abundance, prosperity, and fertility. The celebrations were full of passion and heartfelt glee. Examine your life through these rose-tinted glasses of passion and vitality.

When your heart is in balance, it is easy to flow with grace through both the most mundane and the most challenging actions. Each moment is experienced from a place of neutrality and openness rather than reaction. The trick to this practice isn't squashing down feelings of resentment, sadness, or whatever you are feeling while doing a task. Simply acknowledge what is going on for you. Then you have a choice: If you choose to do something, can you do it with loving intention? Connect with what is really in your heart, and bring that feeling into your work. This is how you create ritual in the mundane.

## SOUL CHALLENGE: *Presence*

In Buddhism there is a practice of washing dishes as if you are wash- ing the baby Buddha. The idea is to treat the thing you are doing as if it is the most important thing in life. You bring a sense of soft joy and gentle care to the task. Choose something you do everyday, such as washing dishes or driving to work. Can you do this task with the same awe, wonder, and reverence you would bring to bathing a sacred baby for the first time?

## GLOBAL APOTHECARY: *Heart Chakra—Anahata*

The heart chakra is the center of all the chakras in the body; there are three chakras above and three below it. The Sanskrit name *anahata* means "unhurt," and relates to the state of being open and free from the wounds of the past. A balanced heart chakra allows you to be open, caring, and forgiving to both yourself and others, with active compassion. The heart chakra is located at the heart and also encompasses the thyroid, the lungs, and the chest generally. Bring your heart chakra into balance by chanting *"yum,"* smiling more, choosing forgiveness, and practicing positive affirmations. Green and pink bring harmony to this chakra.[42]

## Conjuring and Crafting

Now is the magic of the Summer Solstice—time to tune into your dreams, your soul plantings, and your true heart essence, and capture that light to use in the dark seasons. These conjurings elevate mundane ingredients with intention and magic, to soothe and strengthen the heart.

---

### SUMMER SOLSTICE ESSENCE

Invite the power and light from the peak of the season to infuse an essence for you. You can ask a clear quartz crystal to hold the light, as described in Chapter 9, and use flowers in bloom with the glow of the sun, such as dandelions or sunflowers. These suggestions are not prescriptive—feel free to make the essence as nature and intuition guide you.

- Glass bowl
- Piece of cheesecloth or strainer

- Pint-size Mason jar (to store mother essence)
- 1 cup pure spring water or sacred water (water from a holy, pure source)
- Nature item to support your grounding work; if a plant, choose one that is alive and at the peak of its growth, or use a crystal.
- 1 cup organic vodka or brandy

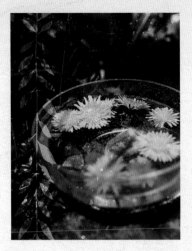

Follow the "Making a Flower Essence" instructions in Chapter 1. Take 1 drop on the tongue, or 3 drops diluted in a glass of water and sipped throughout the day.

---

## LOVE HONEY

This combination of spices, herbs, and flower essences, made with love and pure intention, brings a little brightness and sunshine into dark days.

- 1 jar raw local honey from beloved bees (any size works)
- Zest of 1 orange for a light, joyful heart
- 1 vanilla pod, split open to taste the sweetness in life
- 7 allspice berries, to add the depth of the great mystery
- 1 cinnamon stick, to bring in the spice of the dance
- 3 pieces sun-dried mango, to invite ripe abundance
- 3 drops Summer Solstice Essence (above)

Add all the ingredients to a pot on the stove, and warm them ever-so-gently. *Do not boil.* You are simply using the heat to gently introduce all the spices to the honey. While it is warming, write your intentions on a piece of paper, and read these to your honey.

Place the honey back in the jar, and leave it in a sunny window for a week. Place your written intentions under the jar. After a week, light a candle and read the intentions one more time, then burn the paper to send your intentions up to heaven in the smoke. Finish by saying:

*As it harm none, my will be done.*

*Bless this honey with the light of the sun.*

Strain out the spices, and return the honey to the jar.

Take your honey by the teaspoonful as needed. You could make a couple of jars, and save one for the dark winter nights. It's great for colds—spiritual or otherwise.

---

## SUMMER INCENSE

- 4-ounce jar with lid
- Pestle and mortar
- Clay dish or burner for incense
- 6 Tablespoons powdered sandalwood
- 2 Tablespoons benzoin resin
- 1 Tablespoon elemi resin
- 1 Tablespoon dried rose petals
- 1 Tablespoon nutmeg
- Incense charcoal

Freeze the resins for at least 8 hours before you start. Resins need to be ground with a pestle and mortar, as they tend to gum up and damage grinders. Grind the resins with the nutmeg until the pieces are the size and texture of coarse sea salt.

Remove the resins and nutmeg, and grind the rose petals until fine. Place all ingredients back in the mortar, and grind together to integrate. When well mixed, store them in the jar.

Light your incense charcoal and place in the center of the burner or clay dish. Wait until the charcoal turns gray all over; then place a small scoop of incense on the charcoal. It should make smoke and fragrance. Charcoal needs to breathe, so don't pile too much incense on top of it.

## BONFIRE CEREMONY

Bonfires are a traditional part of Summer Solstice celebrations. Fire is considered purifying, energizing, and warming. It is a wonderful tool for celebration and release work. This ceremony is one way of opening to love and fertility through forgiveness. You need:

- A safe place to have a fire
- A few friends and family you want to share the ceremony with
- Flash paper (This paper burns intensely for a second and then disappears, often found in magic stores.)
- Pens
- Uplifting music

Light the fire, and gather around it. Play a beautiful song while each person considers something they can forgive. It may be directed at themselves—forgiving themselves for not completing a task, for example. Or perhaps it is forgiving another person for a wrong. Forgiveness isn't about saying what happened is okay—it is about choosing to stop giving your energy to that event. When you are ready, write what you are forgiving on the flash paper.

Each person goes around the fire and says something about what they have written. It could be just one word, or a deeper explanation. When they have finished, they throw their flash paper into the fire. Stand back at this point, because the flash paper does flare up. As each person does this, give a cheer, and clap or drum to celebrate the release. When everyone has finished, close the ceremony with eye-smiling. Each person turns to the person next to them, looks that person in the eyes, and smiles.

Now it is time to party. Your hearts are light, the night is young—everybody have some fun! Storytelling and singing together are excellent ways to close the circle.

## Pairings

- Story: "The Golden Deer," a Jataka parable about forgiveness, is great to share with children.
- Class: The Celtic Wheel online class from Sacred Living Movement UK takes you on a fun and meaningful journey through traditional Celtic holidays including solstices and equinoxes.
- Music: "Ancient Light" by Allman Brown is a beautiful song, great for the meditation portion of the bonfire ceremony.

# Journal

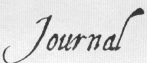

Follow your heart—what do these words
mean to you? Are you living through
compassion and love?

_____

_____

_____

_____

_____

_____

_____

_____

_____

_____

_____

_____

_____

_____

_____

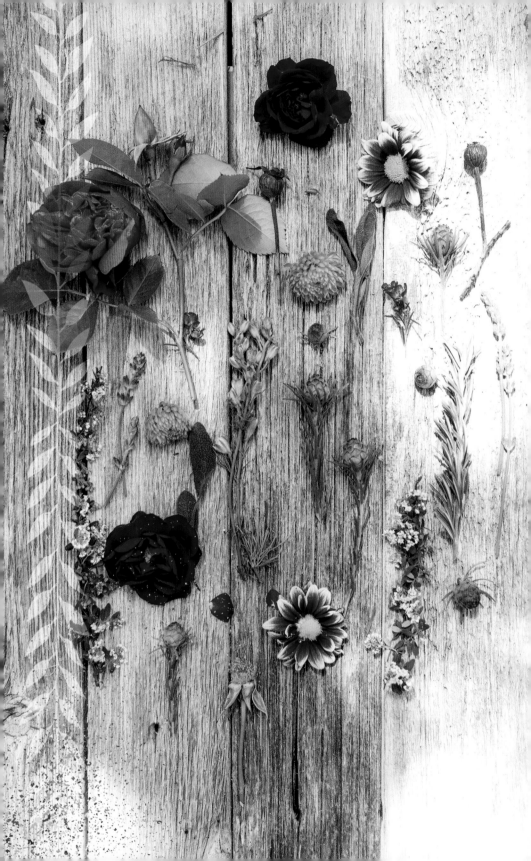

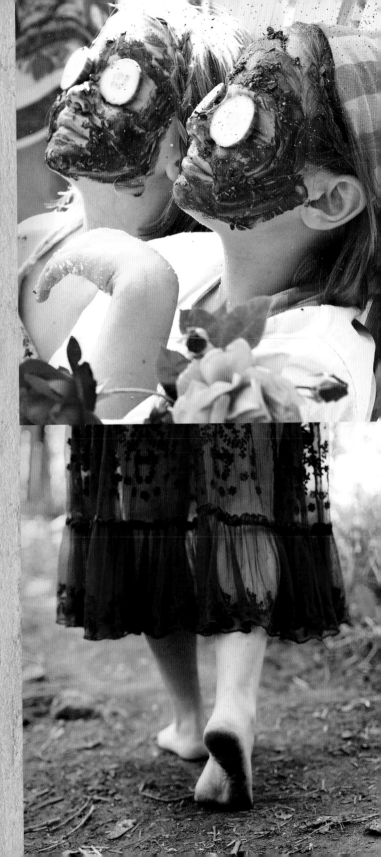

the flower

*emerging teens*

chapter 13

*The fires of the teen years are a crucible for the development of the soul. For many young people, they are the first moments of claiming their sovereignty over their voices, bodies, thoughts, passions, and pains—yet the weighty responsibility of adult reality is still on the horizon. Teen years are spent growing in awareness and connection to the larger community, stepping onto the hero's/heroine's journey path for the first time, and trying on various identities. For teens to truly flower into their best selves, they must have fertile ground to grow, stable space to support wild, inventive behaviors, and open-hearted listening hours available and at the ready.*

## FAMILY WELLNESS: *Hormones*

The physical body of a teenager is in a phase of rapid and relentless growth; the endocrine system kicks into high gear, and hormones take center stage. For teens, regardless of gender, hormones command them to intensely feel everything, and these waves of emotions tend to rule their worlds beyond their control. Learning to moderate these powerful tides comes with maturation, and requires a loving and supportive home life to smooth out emotionally troubled waters.

The endocrine system is incredibly delicate, and works as a feedback system in which one hormone in the chain triggers the next hormone, and so on. Hormones can be thrown out of balance by environmental toxins, poor diet, stress, poor sleep patterns, or illness. Thus, puberty colliding with the lifestyle of Western teenagers creates "perfect storm" conditions. Here are some top tips to gently balance and nourish developing hormone systems.

· **Reduce processed sugar and caffeine consumption.** These wreak havoc on the adrenals and on developing bodies generally.

· **Make rest a priority.** Lack of sleep has been proven to affect testosterone in men and hormones in women.

· **Try a green smoothie or a green supplement.** Green foods remove toxins from the body and nourish the liver. This keeps hormones and body energy flowing smoothly.

- **Take a stress break.** Pressure can inadvertently be put on young people in the home, at school, on social media, and in the larger culture. If teens are not given practices to help them win those internal battles and stay centered, they can easily spiral into emotional pitfalls that are difficult to escape. Listen to your teens, ask questions, be involved in their lives, introduce them to short meditation practices, and provide daily doses of gratitude and living in high vibration so that they have spiritual tools to touch and practice.

- **Talk about sex and intimacy.** It is important to give teens the tools they need to make choices about their fertility and sexual well-being. Talking about sex with your children can be difficult, making people feel awkward and vulnerable, but these discussions are crucial to overall well-being and emotional health. Hormones drive all kinds of emotions and sensations, and sex is certainly one of them. Young people receive so many mixed messages today that talking about healthy body consciousness is essential. Understanding sexual boundaries is necessary to healthy and safe maturation; teaching your teens to value their bodies, so that they are able to receive pleasure, especially from themselves, without feeling shame or guilt promotes healthy sexuality. We do not want our teens to feel pressured into to engaging in sexual behaviors before they are ready, and learning how to truly love themselves is a great way to safeguard against unwanted experiences.

## SPIRITUAL APPLICATION: *Rebellion*

There is a time and a place for rebellion, and it is the job of teens to walk those winding roads. Testing boundaries and exploring freedoms and identities allows for rich soil to be tilled, and fosters greater understanding of their soul's destiny.

This delicate time is when your teens need to be taking risks and learning from their mistakes and triumphs. However, if there are negative self-judgments being played out, or pressure from peers, these soul-stretching leaps can be extra-hard! Allow space in your home for these needed behaviors to flourish and expand. It takes courage to push the boundaries and try something outside your comfort zone at any age—but particularly during this tender developmental teen phase.

## SOUL CHALLENGE: *Rebel*

The stories we often tell ourselves about our worth and abilities in the world can get in the way of being able to claim all of our inner truths and desires. Do you have places within you that have yet to be explored? Have you always wanted to do something that you told yourself you could not accomplish, or are not good enough to succeed at? It's time to wake up your inner rebel, and go for it anyway! Take on one new task this week that stretches you and allows you to take your spirited self on a date, unfolding dormant but lingering desires still living in you.

## GLOBAL APOTHECARY: *Solar Plexus Chakra*

The solar plexus chakra in Sanskrit is called *manipura,* which means "jeweled city" or "lustrous gem." It is associated with the pancreas, liver, and gall bladder, and is located between the navel and the breastbone. It is easy to connect to this chakra by placing your hands in the center of your belly, just under your ribs. Take a deep breath, and see if you can feel a pulse beneath your fingers. This is the beat of the solar plexus chakra.

A balanced third chakra has self-confidence, inner strength, determination, and purpose. Chanting the sound *"ram"* and wearing yellow can help soothe and nourish this chakra into balance. *Manipura* is all about forward motion, and bringing ideas into real life.

## *Conjuring and Crafting*

The best way to get rid of skin blemishes is to prevent them from occurring in the first place. For most people, staying hydrated, eating a whole foods-based diet, and taking care of their hormone health will do this. However, even healthy people can get acne. Here is a face mask to help nourish the skin and soothe blemishes. When using products on your face, do a small patch-test first in a less obvious place such as your arm, to make sure there will be no reaction on your face.

### EDIBLE FACE MASK

- 1 teaspoon raw cocoa powder
- 1 teaspoon fine-milled oats
- 1 teaspoon plain organic yogurt
- 1 teaspoon honey
- 3 drops rose or lotus flower essence

Mix all ingredients together. Apply evenly to your skin. Leave on 10–15 minutes, until dry. When dry, wipe away with warm water. Finish with a cool compress to close the pores, and then a spritz of rosewater or, for dry skin, a light application of rose oil.

Do not use the mask more than once every 10 days.

### KEEP-IT-REAL SPRITZ

This is a deodorant spritzer great to take on the go in your bag or backpack. Many mass-market deodorizing sprays are made with chemicals that disrupt hormones. Feel free to adjust these ingredients by choosing essential oils with fragrances you love.

- 2-ounce spritz bottle
- 2 ounces witch hazel

- 10 drops lemon essential oil
- 10 drops clove essential oil

Mix ingredients together, and fill your spritz bottle. Shake well before use. Spritz under arms and on pulse points as needed. Avoid contact with eyes.

---

## ROSEWATER CLARITY WAND

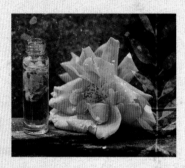

A facial rollerball with sandalwood oil is a good home remedy for clear skin.

- ⅓-ounce (10-ml.) rollerball bottle
- Small bowl for mixing
- Small spoon for stirring
- 21 drops sandalwood essential oil
- 2½ ounces rosewater
- ½ ounce witch hazel

Mix all the ingredients together in the bowl. Stir, and fill the rollerball with your clarity elixir. Roll on face as needed to help clear blemishes.

## Pairings

- Book: *Teenagers: A Natural History* by David Bainbridge—a fun, science-based, and humorous exploration of why the second decade of life is one of the most important.
- Book: *Cycle Savvy: The Smart Teen's Guide to the Mysteries of Her Body* by Toni Weschler. This book is an excellent reference for the young woman who wants to really understand her body.
- Activity: Volunteering at the community level allows teens to explore different people and job opportunities in informal settings.

# Journal

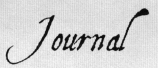

What forgotten part of your inner teen
spirit have you awoken this week?

_____

_____

_____

_____

_____

_____

_____

_____

_____

_____

_____

_____

_____

_____

_____

_____

_____

_____

_____

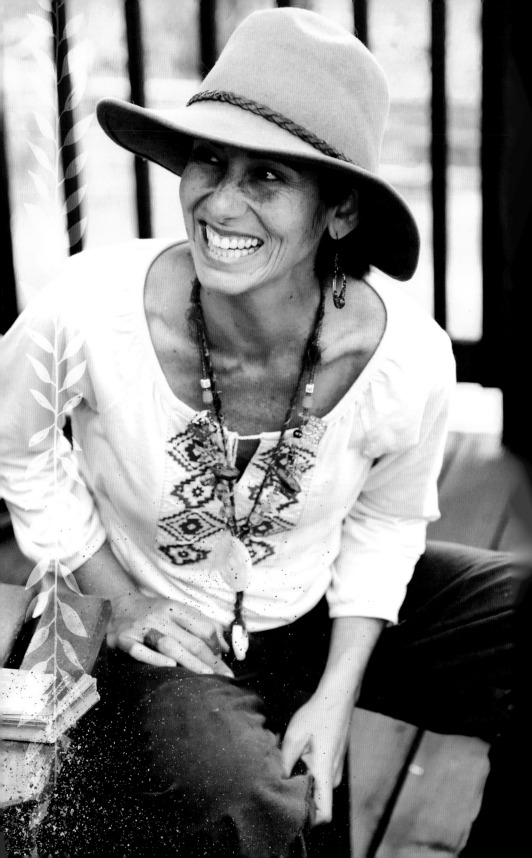

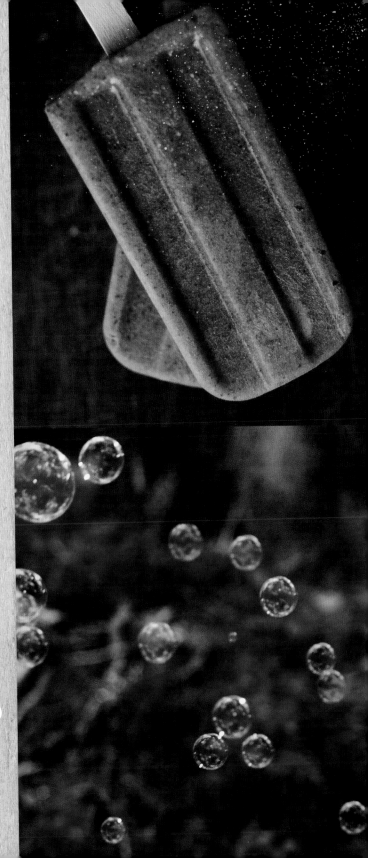

*play*

*laughter is the best medicine*

chapter 14

When there is no pressing agenda or confining task, you can invite more play and bliss into your life. Your children lay the foundation for playtime with an abounding freedom, and if you can release your adult responsibilities for a spell, you can see the world with renewed imagination. Play takes all your skills and unbridles them, luring you into any world you dare to dream up.

## FAMILY WELLNESS: *Laughter Therapy*

Laugh. Go on—do it! And do it out loud. This is something you just have to feel in order to get the full effects of its power. Even the first faltering "Ha! Ha! Ha!" as you get going begins to shake things loose. Laughter is naturally contagious, and you may even find that people near you begin to smile. Laughter is a recognized and well-studied medicinal therapy. When you laugh, not only is your spirit lifted—which you know is key to healing and growth—but physical responses are activated as well. Laughter has been shown to:

· Reduce pain

· Boost both the immune and circulatory systems

· Stimulate the heart and lungs

· Help muscles relax

· Release endorphins

· Improve memory and creativity

· Reduce stress

· Uplift the mood[43]

There are many ways to invite more laughter into your life; playing games, watching funny movies, or simply smiling are all equally effective.[44] You may even consider hosting a family-and-friends comedy night, and give your loved ones a joy-full boost.

### Family comedy night

Give everyone a theme and a time limit for their comedy act. Ask everyone to participate, and ask each person to prepare a few jokes or skits. You could make an evening of it, and start with a silly supper where everyone wears mismatched costumes—zebras with tiaras, or elephants with wings. After dinner, the stage is set for funny-face contests, best-silly-walk contests and, of course, jokes and skits. ·

## SPIRITUAL APPLICATION: *Joy*

Play is a state of being light, spacious, and free. It is often overlooked as the valuable spiritual tool it really is; it can lift you to your highest vibration. It may seem like child's play, but joy is the source of spiritual enlightenment and the key to unlocking nirvana. One of my favorite quotes from Buddha is, *"When you realize how perfect everything is, you will tilt your head back and laugh at the sky."*

## SOUL CHALLENGE: *Inner-Smile Meditation*

A beautiful Taoist and Buddhist practice is called "Inner Smiling," where one focuses attention on inwardly smiling to each part of the body. This practice activates inner compassion and loving-kindness toward yourself and all the major organs in your body.

1. Close your eyes and place your tongue on the roof of your mouth, right behind your front teeth.

2. Create a small smile on your mouth, visualize your heart, and send a loving smile to it for beating and helping you move throughout each day.

3. Proceed to smile to other parts of your body that need attention—particularly to any areas of pain.

4. Extend and share that inner joy and light with the rest of the world.

## GLOBAL APOTHECARY: *Hug Therapy*

Touch is an incredibly comforting and essential part of healing for many people. Hug therapy uses this understanding to support emotional regulation and soothing in times of distress. Consensual, nonsexual touch such as hugging, head-stroking, and hand-holding has been proven to decrease anxiety, panic, and even shame. When done with permission and wholehearted intention, the hug helps the mind and body relax. Next time you are asked for a hug, really commit to it! You are sharing powerful healing.

## *Conjuring and Crafting*

Here is a selection of crafts and food to bring play and delight.

### NATURAL BUBBLES

- Bowl
- Quart-size bottle
- Pipe cleaner
- Selection of beads
- 2 cups liquid castile soap or gentle, organic dish soap
- ½ cup organic sugar
- 5 cups warm water

*To make the bubble mixture:* Mix the sugar in the warm water until it dissolves. Add the soap and mix well. Store in bottle until ready to use.

*To make the bubble wand:* Bend the pipe cleaner in half, and thread a few beads over the two ends. Twist the ends together to hold the beads in place. Pull the top of the cleaner open into a circle to hold the bubble mix.

Dip the wand in the bubble mix, and blow.

## PLAYFUL FEELING MASKS

Make some masks with your children to try on different feelings and perspectives. What happens if you do something in the silly mask? What happens if you do it with the sad mask? The tired mask? The inspired mask? Be creative, and make masks for a wide range of feelings.

- Popsicle sticks
- Paper plates
- Paints, crayons, glitter
- Glue

Cut eyes and mouths in the plates, and decorate them according to the different feelings. Then glue them onto a stick so that you can hold them up to your face.

Take turns pretending to do various tasks, or act out various scenarios wearing the masks.

## CHILDREN'S STORY STONES

Have a playdate out in nature, where you and your little one can find a collection of stones. Ask Mother Earth if you can take them home to use for high-vibration play, and leave a small offering of gratitude—something from nature and your heart.

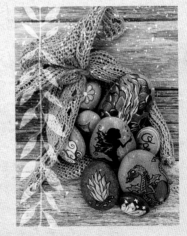

- 6–12 stones
- Paint and brushes
- Your imagination

Choose a picture or symbol for each stone—for example, the elements of Fire, Water, Air, and Earth, or the seasons, favorite animals, a dragon, a princess, an apple, gold, treasure, sword, etc.—and draw or paint one image on each stone. When the paint is dry, turn the stones face-down and scramble them up, or place them all inside a bag.

Then invite imagination into the game. The first person turns over or pulls out one "story stone," and starts a story based on that picture. Then the next person chooses a stone and continues the story with the new image, then the next person, and so on. As the story progresses, take turns choosing stones and adding plot twists. This is a fun way to play with imagination, creativity, and a little help from Mother Nature.

## GREEN MACHINE ICE POPS
*Makes eight 4-ounce pops.*

These Ice Pops are healthy and tasty, and can be used for a treat at a birthday party, or just for playdates with friends.

- 1 cup chopped spinach or kale
- 2 bananas
- 1 whole pineapple, peeled and chopped
- 2 teaspoons chia seeds
- 2 cups purified water

Combine spinach or kale, bananas, and pineapple in blender, and puree. Add chia seeds and water, and puree a second time.

Pour mixture into chosen pop molds, and put sticks in place. Freeze until solid.

*Pairings*

- Book: *Ice Pop Joy* by Anni Daulter
- Flower Essence: Wild strawberry—this flower helps you tap into your wild, sweet, playful nature.
- Book: *The Creative Family: How to Encourage Imagination and Nurture Family Connections* by Amanda Blake Soule

# Journal

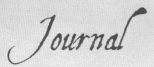

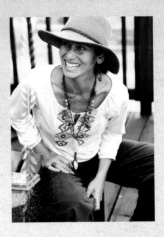

When was the last time you really let go and played—with no worries about the next job on the eternal to-do list of life? Give yourself twenty minutes of play, and then journal here about how you felt before and after.

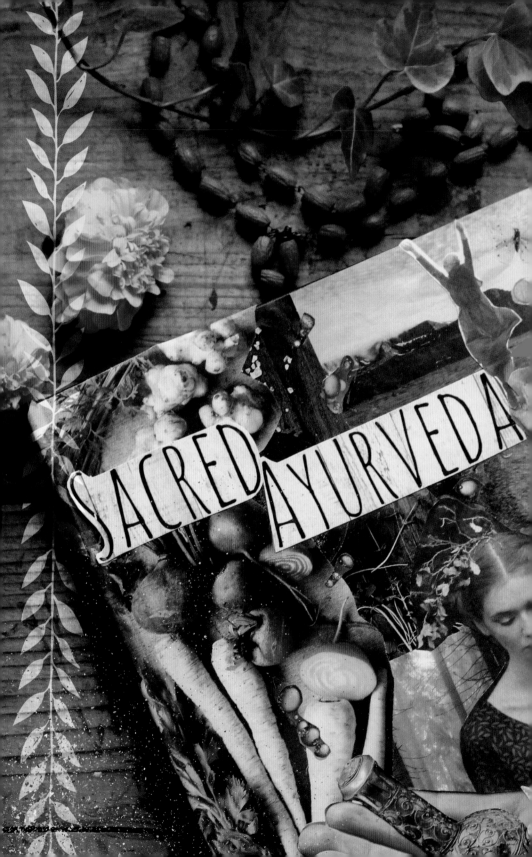

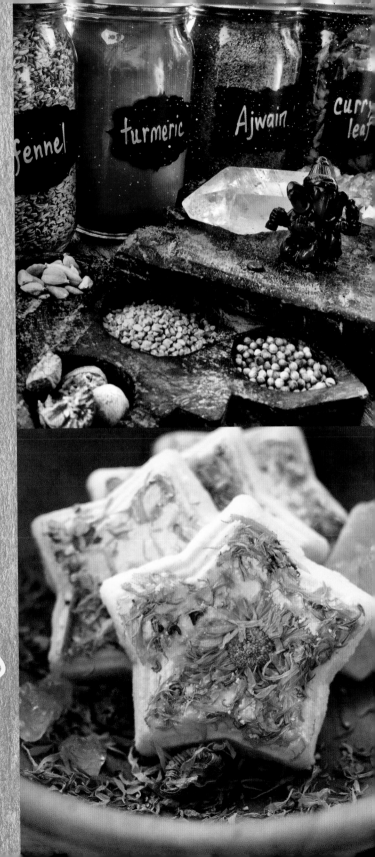

# glow

## the path of selflove

*If you live with passion, love, and integrity, your inner light will glow. Your being is lit by the fires of your soul, and your brilliance shines forth from generously sharing your gifts. Your inner spark is ignited by being loved, witnessed, and nurtured. Conscious care fans the flames of your being, and helps you radiate on all levels with the scintillating shimmer of one who is truly alive.*

## FAMILY WELLNESS: *Skin Health*

The skin is your largest organ. When you are tired, ill, run-down, or out of balance, your skin shows it. Your skin is your first line of defense against germs, and physically shields you from the outside world, yet it is a permeable membrane that takes in nutrients and hydration, and communicates between your inner and outer worlds.

### What are the building blocks of healthy skin?

- A healthy, well-balanced diet
- Good gut health
- Essential fatty acids (EFAs), especially omega 3s
- Vitamins A, C, and E
- The minerals zinc, selenium, and silica

### Looking deeper at essential fatty acids

Essential fatty acids act as hormone regulators, and benefit healthy skin. Omega-3 DHA and omega-6 acids are important structural elements of cell membranes, body tissues, skin, and the brain.

Essential fatty acids need to be in the correct ratio to be bioavailable, and most people get plenty of omega 6 in the Western diet, as this is easily found in vegetable oils. Too much omega 6, however, can stimulate inflammation, which can show on your skin. Omega 3s, to balance the omega 6s, are found in oily fish, flaxseeds, walnuts, and leafy greens.

**Note:** If you are currently taking blood-thinning or blood-sugar medications, talk to your care provider about adding EFAs into your diet.[45]

## SPIRITUAL APPLICATION: *Body-Image Traditions*

While your physical appearance is not the sum of who you are, it makes up much of what is unique about you. Every person's body holds a story with memories that can go back even before you were born. Once you come Earth-side, you begin to spiritually contain those stories within the cells of your body, and your physical environment shapes them into your reality. Take some time to deeply reflect on how you experience and see your physical body—is it your temple?

*How do you take care of your body and talk to yourself about it?*

The light of your soul illuminates you from within, and your confidence and awareness define your brand of beauty. Develop a powerful vocabulary for describing yourself to others that encompasses love and respect. The subtle ways you talk about "you" and your own beauty spill over into the consciousness of the people around you, so be sure to send the right message about how you feel about yourself.

## SOUL CHALLENGE: *Body Prayer*

A body prayer is a series of movements done with the intention to connect with the divine source of life.

Reach up and gather in the light of heaven, and with hand gestures wash the glittering light over your body. Breathe deep, reach down with more hand gestures, and sweep the molten gold from Earth's core into your body. Breathe deep again, and state, *"I am a child of light, a guardian of Earth, and a supremely divine being."* Wrap your arms around yourself, and hug your heart.

## GLOBAL APOTHECARY: *Ayurveda*

Ayurveda is a 5,000-year-old traditional Indian medicine practice rooted in observation of the human body, mind, and soul. It sees
the whole person not as a series of symptoms but as an expression of
energy. It is founded on the idea that mind and body are deeply connected. Being in balance allows you to live to your fullest potential.
Ayurveda uses herbs, diet, movement, and massage to nurture this
balance.

## Conjuring and Crafting

### AYURVEDIC BODY OIL

*A simple luxury for glowing skin, this recipe is generously shared
by Radha Schwaller, Ayurvedic practitioner with Bliss Alchemy.*

Oiling the skin in Ayurveda is called *snehana* in Sanskrit. This
means "oil therapy," and is also LOVE therapy. Anointing the
skin daily with loving intentions using high-quality oil made by
you is one of the most simple and luxurious things you can do
for your health.

- 2 ounces calendula (*Calendula officinalis*)-infused jojoba oil
  (see "Infused Oils" instructions in Chapter 4 for this and
  the following infused oils)
- 1 ounce rose-infused jojoba oil
- ½ ounce elderflower-infused jojoba oil
- ½ ounce *shatavari* (*Asparagus racemosus*)-infused jojoba oil
- 10 drops geranium essential oil, for fertility, health, protection, and love
- 10 drops frankincense essential oil, for pure spiritual
  connection

- 6 drops tulsi essential oil, for spiritual abundance and clarity of mind
- 10 drops vetiver essential oil, for connecting to the Earth and relieving worry
- 6 drops Himalayan cinnamon essential oil, for prosperity
- 8 drops lemon essential oil (use steam-distilled to avoid phototoxicity), to uplift the spirit

Mix infused oils together and stir gently. Add essential oils one at a time, gently stirring between additions. Store in a labeled amber or blue glass bottle for up to one year.

## HOW TO PERFORM A SELF-MASSAGE
### (Abhyanga)

Remember you are anointing your body with oil as a way of loving yourself, and to enhance your health in mind, body, and spirit. Take your time, and be gentle and soft with yourself.

1. Gently heat your massage oil. Warm the oil in its container by placing the bottle in a sink or bowl full of warm water.

2. Begin by applying a small amount of oil to the top of your head. Massage the top of the head in a clockwise manner with the center of your palm. This is one of the maha marma ("great secret") points, and regulates the amount of prana, or life-force energy, that moves throughout the body.

3. Apply oil to the entire body, beginning with the neck and arms. Remember to use circular motions over the joints, and long strokes on the limbs.

4. Make clockwise circular strokes around the breast area and on the abdominal area.

5. Continue the sequence to the hips, buttocks, and legs, ending with the feet.

6. Let the oil soak in for 5–20 minutes, depending on your timeframe. Be sure to stay out of drafts and in a warm space during this time.

7. Take a warm bath or shower. Use gentle soap only where needed; it is good if a little oil remains on the skin.

8. Repeat daily.

## WHIPPED MANGO BODY BUTTER

Mango Body Butter is a creamy, nourishing blend that soaks right into your skin. To get a good fluffy texture, keep the proportions at ¾ solid ingredients and ¼ liquid, and make sure it has cooled enough before you start whipping.

- ½ cup mango butter
- ½ cup cocoa butter
- ½ cup coconut oil
- ¼ cup almond oil
- ¼ cup mango seed oil (this is kinda pricey, so feel free to substitute plain almond oil or a favorite infused oil)
- 20 drops of your favorite essential oil (optional)

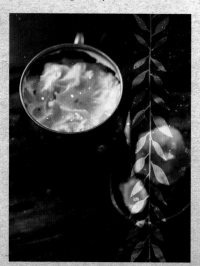

Melt together all the ingredients except the essential oil in a double-boiler, stirring well. Once well combined, remove the mixture from the heat and allow to cool a little; then add the essential oils.

Cool the mix thoroughly, until it begins to solidify. Now is the time to whip! Using a hand mixer is easiest, and takes about 10–15 minutes.

If you live in a hot climate, this is best kept in a cool place. Otherwise, room temperature is fine. Rub lovingly into your skin, as you like.

## ROSE SHIMMER CREAM

- ½ cup shea butter
- ½ cup cocoa butter
- ½ cup coconut oil
- ½ cup infused rose petal oil (see "Infused Oils" instructions in Chapter 4)
- 3 teaspoons gold or pink mica
- 20 drops of rose essential oil

Melt all the ingredients together, except the essential oil and mica, in the top of a double-boiler (or in a glass bowl set on a pan of gently boiling water), stirring well. Once well combined, remove the mixture from the heat, allow it to cool a little, and then add the essential oils.

Now cool the mix thoroughly. It should be starting to solidify. Now is the time to whip it! Using a hand mixer is the easiest way to accomplish this. Once it starts to gain volume, add the mica and keep whipping, for about 10–12 minutes.

If you live in a hot climate, this is best kept in a cool place. Otherwise, room temperature is fine. Rub lovingly into your skin, as you like.

## SUMMER BATH BOMBS

- Large measuring jug
- Round dome molds, plastic eggs, silicon cupcake cups/tray, or similar molds
- 1 cup baking soda
- ½ cup citric acid

- ½ cup organic cornstarch
- ½ cup fine Epsom salt
- 1–2 teaspoons water
- 1 teaspoon natural coconut extract
- ½ teaspoon sandalwood essential oil
- ½ teaspoon rose essential oil
- 1 teaspoon almond oil, or your favorite infused oil
- Dried organic calendula petals

Mix all the dry ingredients except calendula petals in a bowl. Mix all the wet ingredients in a measuring jug. Prepare your molds by placing a teaspoon of dried calendula petals at the bottom of each one.

Ever so slowly, pour the wet ingredients into the dry ingredients, and incorporate them together. Test-scoop some of the mixture out, and see if it holds together; if it doesn't, add a tiny bit more water. Go slowly! Too much water can spoil the batch. (If you do add too much water, all is not lost—just pour it all into a jar, and add a spoonful at a time to the bath instead of forming it into balls.) Once the mixture is holding together, pack it firmly into your molds, pressing it into the calendula petals. If using two-sided molds, pack both sides full, then press them together.

Now you need some patience. Let them dry for about 15–20 minutes, then very gently remove them from the molds. Place them on wax paper to harden for about 24 hours.

Add 1 or 2 bombs to the bath. They store well in an airtight jar or container.

## Pairings

- Supplements: Nordic Naturals has an excellent range of omega-fat supplements.

- Plant Ally: Evening primrose—the unsaturated fatty acid and gamma linoleic acid in evening primrose balances skin and hormones.

- Class: "Sacred Ayurveda" explores your *dosha* (mind/body type) to bring harmony and balance to your daily life.

# Journal

What power words can you use to describe your glow? What gifts are you sharing with the world?

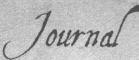

_____

_____

_____

_____

_____

_____

_____

_____

_____

_____

_____

_____

_____

_____

_____

_____

_____

_____

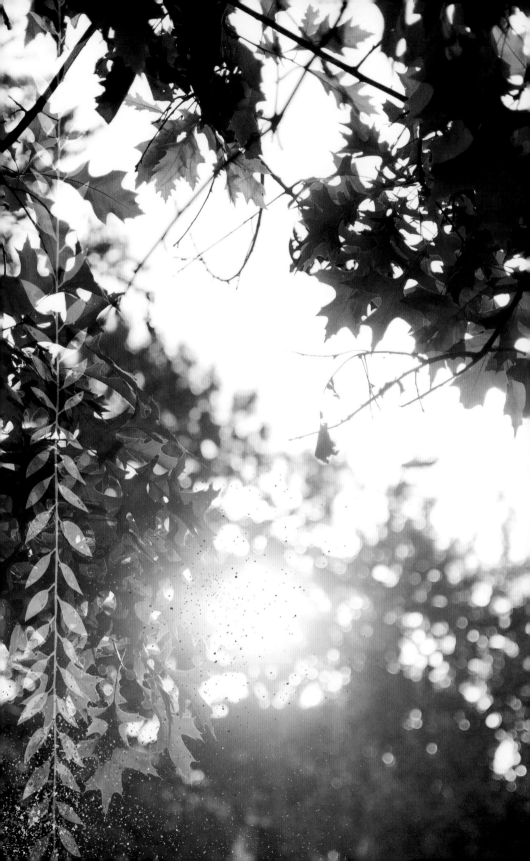

the sun

*what the day knows*

chapter 16

*You contain in every cell the light of the sun. You are the incandescence of stars, and you shine. The sun is the vibrant yang to the moon's yin. It is the dance; it is the laughter; it is the passion. Sun power is your own potent action, your own brightest burst. The sun feeds you on every level with the spark of the heavens. You feel this nourishment everywhere, in your roots and in the depths of your soul. You thrive.*

## FAMILY WELLNESS: *The Sun and Vitamin D*

The sun intrinsically feeds our cells. The stimulating power of sunlight catalyzes the formation of the essential nutrient vitamin D. Researchers discovered that the T cells of the immune system use vitamin D as part of their activation process. Without functioning T cells, the body cannot fight off infections and viruses. Vitamin D is also an essential component of the endocrine system, and helps with calcium homeostasis in the cells of the body.

Humans are able to synthesize vitamin D with exposure to sunlight.[46] However, this is a dance to perform with caution. Too much time in the sun can lead to burns, dehydration, sunstroke, or even skin cancer. This is a call for balancing good sense with real-life practice.

### Good sun practices

- **Avoid the sun** at the hottest part of the day (usually after noon, depending on where you are).
- **Wear sensible clothing.** Hats, sunglasses, and light, loose clothing all offer protection.
- **Use a good-quality, natural sun cream** with SPF 15 or higher. Buyer beware—many popular conventional brands are full of carcinogenic chemicals. This is an area worth doing some extra research.
- **Seek shade,** and remember that if your skin feels very hot, that is a sign of burning, and you are being exposed to UV radiation.

## SPIRITUAL APPLICATION: *Accomplishment*

A big part of spiritual wellness is a sense of accomplishment. Are you doing what you came here to do? Are you shining your light—as big and bright as it can be? You are a part of this divine creation, and you are worthy to be here. *Bask in the golden glory of the sun,* and infuse this light into every molecule of your being.

## SOUL CHALLENGE: *Sun Energy*

Hold your hands up to the sun, and feel the light collecting in your cupped palms. Breathe in deeply, and imagine you are inhaling the sunlight. As you inhale, your ribs and belly expand, full of this warm glow. As you exhale, breathe out the beautiful light all around you. Continue this practice until you are positively humming, full of light, surrounded by light. Now pick a small achievable goal—and do it! Don't wait till you are ready or everything is perfect. Choose this moment to take the first step in activating your creative, expressive self.

## GLOBAL APOTHECARY: *Sun Magick*

Sun magick is the practice of using the sun to activate and charge your intentions and work. Sunlight can also be used to clean crystals. The underlying energy is one of activation, ambition, achievement, and ascension. Sun magick is great for any work that calls for growth, expansion, enlightenment, and power.

## Conjuring and Crafting

---

### NATURAL SUN PROTECTION LOTION

*Makes about 5 ounces. Our sweet friend and talented herbalist Sarah Josey from Golden Poppy Herbal Apothecary in Fort Collins, CO, has shared one of her tried and tested homemade sun-cream recipes.*

- 2-cup Pyrex measuring cup
- Pan for hot water
- Stirring implement
- Sifter
- Jar for storing final product
- Label
- 2 ounces shea butter
- 2 ounces coconut oil
- ½ ounce beeswax
- ½ ounce grapeseed oil
- 1 ounce zinc powder
- Optional—essential oils, for scent; do not use citrus essential oils, as these are photosensitizing and will make the cream less effective

Place shea butter, coconut oil, beeswax, and grapeseed oil in the top of a double-boiler, or in a measuring cup placed in a pan of water on the stove. Heat until all of the solids have melted together. Sift in the zinc powder, and stir well to incorporate. Add any essential oils that you may want to include at this time. While still melted, pour into a glass jar for stor-

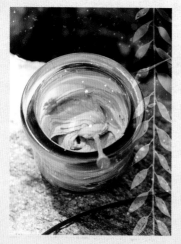

age. Allow to cool in a protected place, without the lid on. Label the jar.

Apply to skin before going out in the sun. It may need reapplication after 40 minutes to 2 hours, depending on the person's skin type and the outdoor activity level.

**Note:** This cream will melt if kept in a hot car or directly in the sun, so it's best to keep it in a cool place. It will re-harden, but may need a good stir if this happens.

This cream is water- and sweat-resistant.

---

## LIP BALM

- 8 lip balm containers (about ⅛ ounce each)
- ¼ cup red raspberry seed oil
- ¼ cup cocoa butter
- ¼ cup beeswax
- 20 drops of rose, sweet orange, or vanilla essential oil (optional)
- 1 teaspoon mica for color (optional)

Gently melt the oil and cocoa butter in a double-boiler or a heatproof glass bowl set over a pan of simmering water. Add beeswax, and stir until it is all melted.

Remove from heat, and allow to cool a little before adding remaining ingredients. Pour into desired containers. It will harden as it cools.

---

## AFTER-SUN BALM

A soothing and cooling balm for tender skin after a day in the sun.

- 8-ounce Mason jar
- double-boiler (or heatproof glass bowl set over a pan of gently boiling water)
- ½ cup infused oil (see "Infused Oils" instructions in Chapter 4)
- ¼ cup aloe vera gel
- ⅛ cup beeswax

- 3 drops blue lotus or self-heal flower essence
- 20 drops essential oil—choose among these:

*Geranium*—cooling, uplifting, very soothing for burns and redness

*Chamomile*—soothing for skin conditions, calming

*Lavender*—soothing for skin conditions, calming

*Frankincense*—cooling and healing

*Sandalwood*—cooling and healing

Melt the infused oil, calendula oil, aloe vera gel, and beeswax in a double-boiler (or heatproof bowl set on a pan of boiling water). Remove from heat, and mix in essential oil and flower essences.

Place in clean glass jar to cool. Use topically as needed.

## Pairings

- Plant Ally: Aloe vera—place in your medicine cupboard and ask it to keep all your creations at a high, pure vibration. Use when needed.
- Music: "I am the Black Gold of The Sun" by Nuyorican Soul—expressive, lifting, smooth. The perfect expansive sun song.
- Website: Environmental Workings Groups Annual Sunscreen Guide—check out this online guide to the best ready-made natural sunblocks; it is updated every year, and very comprehensive: www.ewg.org/sunscreen/
- Movement: Yoga Sequence—Sun Salutation. Learn this movement sequence in online videos, or any yoga class. It gets the body moving, creating a sensation of warmth and vitality.

# Journal
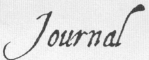

How do you foster a sense of accomplishment in yourself and in others? Take some
time to explore the quality of your light.

_____

_____

_____

_____

_____

_____

_____

_____

_____

_____

_____

_____

_____

_____

_____

_____

_____

_____

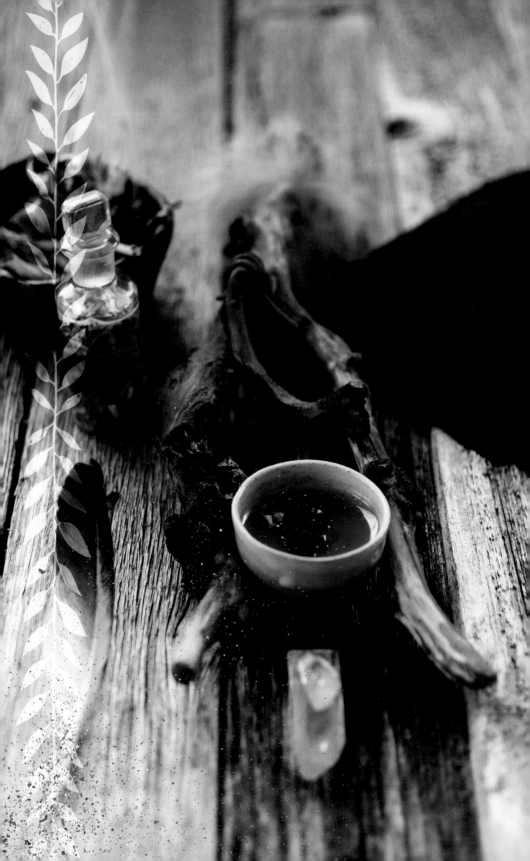

# wings

*praying & receiving*

_____

chapter 17

What do you need to nourish it?

*You have spiritual wings that unfurl when needed, even if you cannot see them. They are the wings that hold you up, give you hope, help you soar to heights you never knew possible, and connect you to the Divine. You are first spirit and soul, and then body—although we tend to mix those up here on Earth. We must honor the physical, earthy body, but without our spiritual wings in working order, we can't easily fly.*

## FAMILY WELLNESS: *Your Body Is Your Temple*

Your body is the material home of your soul. It is part of you, but does not define the totality of your existence. Your body has its own innate wisdom, and deserves to be listened to. When you approach your body with neutral listening, you are gifted with its stories.

When you are ill, it can be so difficult to have this kind of patience and tolerance for your body. However, being sick is not your body's fault. Be aware of how your inner self-talk and outer care reflect your feelings about your body. Your body is the temple of your soul, and thrives when you adorn it with reverence.

One way to enter into communion with your body and soul is through praying. Praying is medicine for the spirit. It is a powerful and underused tool in today's world. There is research showing that prayers do have a positive effect on health and wellness.[47] Do not be afraid of your invisible wings—they have the power to carry you farther than you know.

## SPIRITUAL APPLICATION: *Your Divinity*

You are sacred, precious, and worthy, and the uniqueness of your being is irreplaceable. There has never been another you, and there never will be. This isn't ego-fueled narcissism, but an acknowledgment of your intrinsic divinity. Your divinity is a real experience, not a mysterious theory. Many sacred texts from all over the world refer to this inner light or God-spark. Regularly touching this place inside of you, through prayer and meditation, helps you authentically live out your purpose. It puts you in alignment with your highest calling and your truest medicine.

## SOUL CHALLENGE: *The Art of Blessing and Praying*

The art of praying, or adding blessings and gratitude to your daily life, is a gift we are all granted and can tap at any moment. You can never imprison the free soul. Take up many ways of using this medicine gift in your life, and see what effects it has on you and your family. When you bless your food, your water, your garden, and your family, you are awakening their inner divinity. When you pray, you commune with the greater divinity of the universe. Hone your fine prayer skills by practicing them every day for a week. Find a way to do them that is authentic and speaks from your soul.

## GLOBAL APOTHECARY: *Crown Chakra*

The crown chakra is located at the top of the head. It is the gateway to our connection with the Divine Spirit. Its name, *sahasrara*, means "the thousand-petaled lotus," and symbolizes enlightenment. When the crown chakra is open and in balance, you are able to let go of ego and step into expansive awareness. The sound *"om"* and the color violet help to balance this chakra.[48]

## *Conjuring and Crafting*

---

### DIVINE WISDOM POTION

This is a delightful potion to encourage insight and connection to divine wisdom.

- 1 cup apple juice
- 1 cinnamon stick—a "wand of knowing"

- 1 star anise—for the mystery of the cosmos
- 1 clear quartz—for the memory of the Earth
- 1 teaspoon honey—"golden bee elixir"
- 3 drops essence from a wise tree; we like to use pine, yew, or willow

Mix all ingredients in a saucepan on medium heat until warm. Do not boil. Turn off heat, and let steep for 10 minutes. Say this spell:

*Divine Wisdom within,*

*Divine Wisdom outside,*

*I call upon you to*

*Awaken and speak to my Inner Guide.*

Strain out spices, and drink your potion. Use it to help with inspiration and creative thinking.

---

## TRANQUILITY ESSENCE

Try your hand at making an essence that will help you tap into your tranquil divinity. Choose a tree, plant, or crystal that calls to your heart. Ask Mother Nature for what you most need, and she will answer.

- Glass bowl
- Piece of cheesecloth, or strainer
- Pint-size Mason jar (to store mother essence)
- 1 cup pure spring water or sacred water (water from a holy, pure source)
- A nature item to support your tranquil divinity; if a plant, choose materials when alive and at the peak of their growth
- 1 cup organic vodka or brandy

If using flowers, follow the instructions in Chapter 1 for "Making a Flower Essence."

Take 1 drop on the tongue, or 3 drops diluted in a glass of water and sipped through the day.

---

## WINGS AND PRAYERS CEREMONY

Send your prayers to the heavens on the wings of a feather.

- A found feather from nature
- Your prayers
- A small gratitude offering—for example, strands of your hair, a crystal, fresh water, organic compost, or birdseed

Ask Mother Nature to help you find a feather. Leave your gratitude offering in thanks for the feather. Find a quiet place to sit. Whisper your prayers to the feather, with heartfelt words and truth.

When you are ready, blow vacross the feather to gift the prayers with your divine breath of life. Release the feather back to nature and the heavens, sending your prayers out into the world.

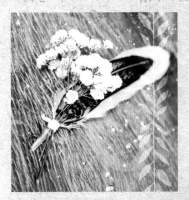

### Pairings

- Plant Ally: Angelsword—this essence helps you hear the words of angels, and protects your energy fields from harm.
- Crystal: Blue chalcedony—a radiant stone that helps you connect to the angelic realms, and supports meditation and stability.
- Resource: *Guardian Angel Tarot Cards* by Doreen Virtue and Radleigh Valentine—a comforting and sweet tarot deck based on angels.

# Journal

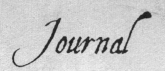

What kind words would your guardian
angel say to you right now?

_____

_____

_____

_____

_____

_____

_____

_____

_____

_____

_____

_____

_____

_____

_____

_____

_____

_____

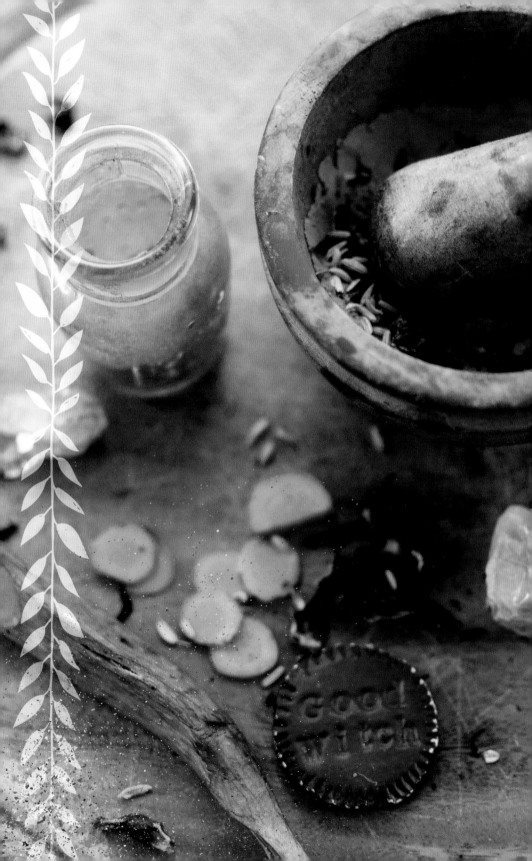

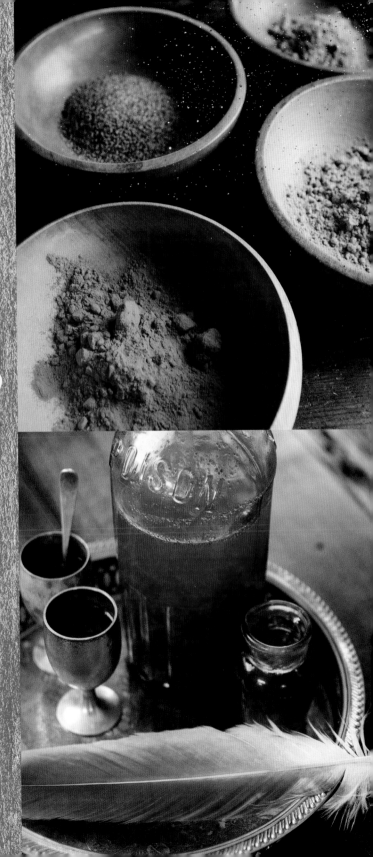

*alchemy*

*activating healing*

chapter 18

*Alchemy is the archaic practice of transforming matter from one state to another—base metal to gold, rocks to jewels, or humble plants into a universal healing elixir. It is the activation of the hidden intrinsic power that resides in everyone and everything. Rouse your inner mystic; stoke the flames of inspiration and creativity. Reveal your inner gold, and live to the fullest.*

## FAMILY WELLNESS: *Spice it Up*

Asian medicine traditions have long used spices to aid in nourishing health and well-being. Spices are alluring, mysterious, and healing. Recent studies are supporting this tantalizing practice, and the even better news is that many of the spices can benefit you just from eating a small amount of them in a day. Enliven your being with potent aromatics like these:

**Cinnamon** can be used as a sweet or savory spice. Ceylon cinnamon is the healthiest because it has a lower concentration of the compound coumarin, which can be harmful in large doses. Make sure to check your labels when buying. Even at two teaspoons per day, cinnamon has been shown to have many benefits.

*Properties of cinnamon* are anti-inflammatory, antioxidant, antibacterial, and antifungal. It has been known to lower and stabilize blood sugar in both Type 1 and Type 2 diabetes. Cinnamon can also improve the ratio of LDL ("bad") to HDL ("good") cholesterol, and has been known to have beneficial effects on neurodegenerative diseases including Alzheimer's and Parkinson's.[49]

**Ginger** is a root that can be used fresh, dried, or powdered. It can be a sweet or savory spice, and adapts well to many recipes.

*Properties of ginger* are anti-inflammatory, antioxidant; can reduce some types of nausea and vomiting; has been known to lower blood sugar, reduce factors that contribute to heart disease, and relieve chronic indigestion and menstrual and muscle pain. Ginger is also known to reduce LDL (bad) cholesterol, enhance brain functions such as reaction time and working memory, and is also antibacterial and antiviral.[50]

**Cayenne** is a thin, red pepper found in Southern, Mexican, and Asian traditions. It can be used fresh, dried, or powdered, and it packs a hot punch in any recipe.

*Properties of cayenne* are antibacterial, antifungal; can break up mucus, or act as a digestive aid and circulatory stimulant; supports detoxification; can prevent factors that lead to blood clots; can be a joint-pain reliever and metabolic activator.[51, 52]

**Garlic** has near-legendary status as a cure-all—and for good reason. This spice has been used for centuries to boost overall health and treat illness. It can be enjoyed roasted, fresh, dried, powdered, and smashed.

*Properties of garlic* are antioxidant, antibacterial, antiviral; can boost the immune system, and is nutrient-rich with vitamins C and B6, manganese, selenium, and other minerals. Garlic can reduce blood pressure, improve cholesterol levels, and help detoxify the body of heavy metals.[53]

### Get your spice on!

Add cinnamon and ginger to your breakfast cereal and desserts, and mix them into teas, coffees, and hot chocolates. Make a cayenne-garlic-ginger spice blend to add to stir-fries, salad dressings, and sauces.

Adding spices to your diet through food should not be a problem in terms of health and digestion. However, these spices contain powerful compounds, so if you are taking medications you need to check with your care provider. Large supplemental quantities of these spices could interfere with prescriptions.

## SPIRITUAL APPLICATION: *Creation and Destruction*

An inventor does not wait until all conditions are perfect to begin working. Sometimes you just have to dive into the throes of your creative forces, and realize that you may not strike gold every time—and that is okay. Being brave enough to take a chance on an idea is how you make something new, exciting, and something that nobody has ever seen before. This magical process can end in a giant mess, where everything must get torn apart several times and rebuilt anew, where your hypothesis does not always work out, and where you put your heart and soul into a vision that only you can still see as needed and perfect. So be it. Surrender to the chaos of the flying leap, and turn that base metal of your being into something brilliant.

## SOUL CHALLENGE: *Get Activated*

Think of something you have always wanted to do but have been delaying due to timing, money concerns, or fear. Write a list of three steps you need to take to achieve that goal. Great! Now take the first step.

## GLOBAL APOTHECARY: *Subtle Bodies*

"Subtle bodies" is the name given to define the many layers of the human being beyond the *physical body*, which is concrete, grounded, and material. All of the subtle bodies are rooted in the physical body, which means that they are part of and connected to the physical body.

The first layer is the *etheric body*. This part contains the aura, the meridians of Traditional Chinese Medicine, and the chakras of Ayurvedic practice. Many people have tangible and visual experiences of the etheric body through bodywork, meditation, and intuition. The second layer is referred to as the *astral body*. This body is interactive, fluid, and conscious. All feelings, sensations, images, and interactions, both in the physical plain and on the astral plane, influence this field. This is the home of memory, intellect, imagination, and determination. Finally, there is the *spiritual body*, which is the divine blueprint of the soul. It is the place that connects the individual soul with the unity of the Source (the Divine).

# Conjuring and Crafting

## FIRE CIDER (MASTER'S TONIC)

Fire Cider, also known as Master's Tonic, is full of beneficial spices, and is the ultimate *hot and spicy* tonic to really get the body energy moving. As our herbalist friend Sarah Josey says, whichever you way you make Fire Cider is the right way. This is a classic recipe, made and adapted through the ages.

- Quart-size glass jar
- 1 cup fresh horseradish, peeled and chopped
- 1 cup chopped yellow onion
- 1 cup fresh garlic, peeled
- ½ cup fresh ginger, peeled and chopped
- ½ cup fresh turmeric, peeled and chopped
- 1–3 fresh chili peppers (to your taste)
- ¼–½ teaspoon cayenne powder (to your taste)
- 1 quart raw apple cider vinegar
- ¼–½ cup raw local honey (to taste)

Chop all the roots into roughly similar-size pieces. Pack the horseradish, onion, and garlic into the jar. Add fresh ginger and fresh turmeric. The jar should be about ⅔ full.

Pour in the raw apple cider vinegar to cover everything by 2–3 inches. Pack in the fresh chilis, or a sprinkle of cayenne. Since this tonic rests for 4 weeks, the spice really permeates, so beware—a little goes a long way!

Cover tightly and leave to work its magic for 4 weeks. Then strain the veggies out and gift them to your compost with gratitude.

Mix the liquid with raw local honey to taste. Fire Cider is best when it tastes hot, spicy, and sweet. Take a shot a day to keep colds away. This is perfect for cold conditions where symptoms include white or clear runny snot, chills, aches, and pains.

Fire Cider can also be added at the end of cooking to sauces or steamed vegetables, or to salad dressings and soups.

---

## CAYENNE AND GINGER ANTI-INFLAMMATORY SALVE

*Makes about 8 ounces. This recipe is shared by herbalist Sarah Josey at Golden Poppy Herbal Apothecary in Fort Collins, CO.*

- Large glass Mason jar
- Disposable medical gloves
- Eye protection
- Double-boiler
  (or heatproof glass bowl set on a pan of gently boiling water)
- Crockpot
- Large pan
- Cheesecloth
- Wooden stirring stick
- Jars or tins for finished salve
- Labels and pens
- ½ ounce St. John's wort
- ½ ounce dried ginger root
- ¼ ounce cayenne pepper
- 8 ounces olive oil
- 1 ounce beeswax
- Optional—essential oils of your choice. We like juniper and rosemary, but any of the anti-inflammatory/pain-relieving oils would work well. Be sure to follow safety and dilution guidelines for all essential oils.

Place the herbs in a large Mason jar, and shake well to mix. Cover the herbs with the olive oil, and stir well. Place the lid on the jar, and place the jar in a water bath in a crockpot set on low for 12 hours, to allow the herbs to infuse into the oil.

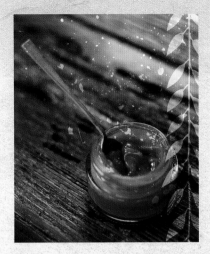

Strain the oil through cheesecloth into the top of a double-boiler (or into a Pyrex measuring cup), squeezing out as much oil as possible. **Note:** Wear disposable medical gloves and perhaps eye protection during this part, as any amount of cayenne-infused oil in your eyes would be very painful and possibly damaging.

Add the beeswax to the oil, and heat the double-boiler on the stove (or place the measuring cup into a pan of hot water on the stove). Heat until the beeswax is melted. Add any essential oils you choose.

Pour into jars or tins, and label them after the salve has cooled and hardened.

## Pairings

- Resource: Frontier Natural Foods Co-op is a great place to order a wide variety of spices (www.frontiercoop.com)
- *Cookbook: The Spice Merchant's Daughter* by Christina Arokiasamy—a beautifully written book full of family history and satisfying recipes.

# Journal

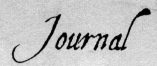

Explore your alchemical skills this week. Experiment with spices, activate your dreams, and transmute base materials. How are you pushing the boundaries of your soul with these tasks?

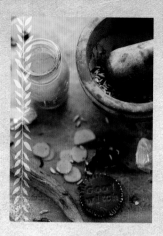

_____

_____

_____

_____

_____

_____

_____

_____

_____

_____

_____

_____

_____

_____

_____

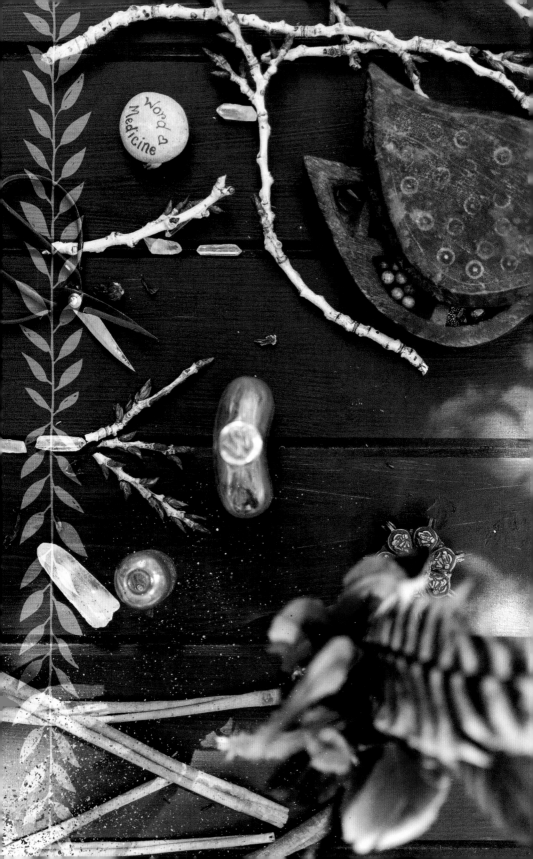

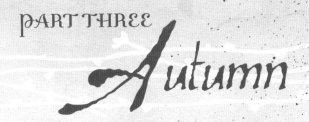

# PART THREE

# Autumn

Come, Dear Ones, Autumn calls.

The siren song of the shapeshifter invites you home.

Listen to the stories of ancient crows,

Whispered into the rising wind.

Bask, full and sensual, in ripe languor.

The harvest glow of contentment and

The sweet heart-song of gratitude imbues the air.

Now is the velvet, dusky softness of the twilight—

We slow-dance with the mystery of the beckoning long dark.

Come to the edge with me, Dear Ones,

Berry-stained fingers tracing beloved lips,

The smell of wood smoke in long, flowing hair,

The crackling of leaves under bare feet,

The mist of warm breath coiling around us.

The Dark Season draws near.

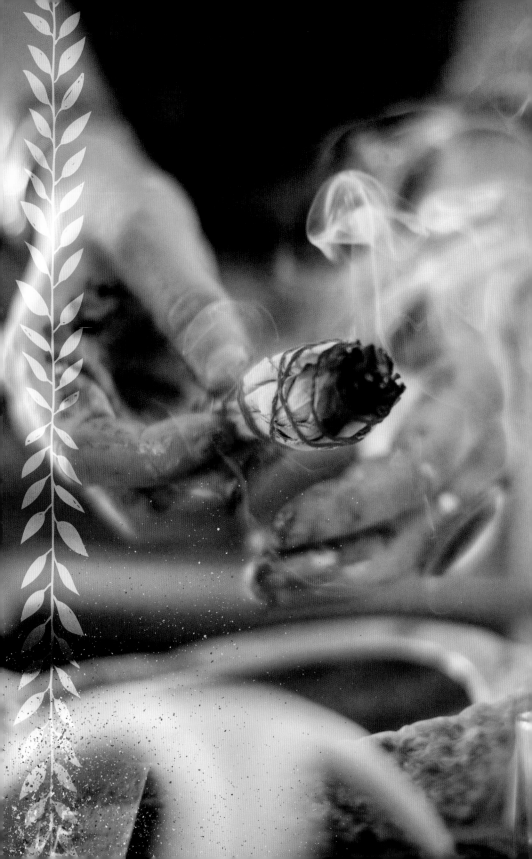

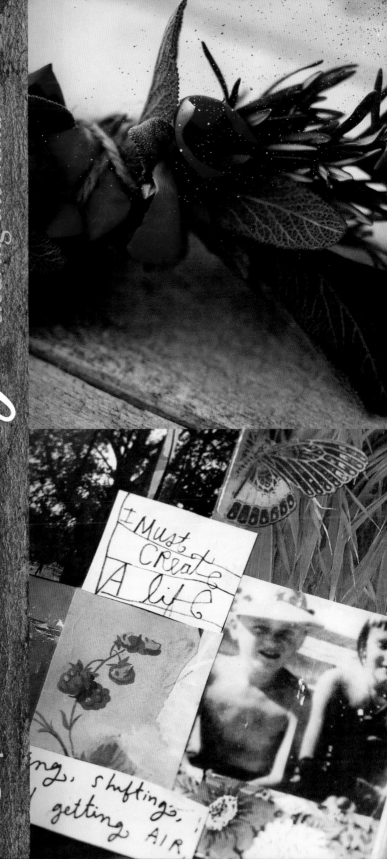

# twilight
*clearing the mind*

chapter 19

*Walking in the half-light where the last of the sun's rays cling to the edges of the land, a burning ember against the inky curtain of the night sky softly lights your truth. In this place you gaze on transformation. It is a gateway from one state to another—summer shimmers into fall, children return for another year, older and wiser, to the studies of school, and the magical power of twilight is everywhere. You hear the siren call of the shape-shifting season. Follow it.*

## FAMILY WELLNESS: *Nourishing the Mind*

Brain health is essential, no matter what your age. Caring for concentration and memory is important not just for school children but also for adults, especially over the age of thirty. The easiest way to stimulate health in a brain is to use it—challenging yourself to engage with life, learn new information, try novel activities, and develop fresh skills creates new neural pathways and changes old patterns and connections. This ability of nerve tissue to adapt is called *neuroplasticity.*[54]

### Worry and overthinking

In Traditional Chinese Medicine, worry and overthinking are causes of disease. This connection is backed up by recent research indicating that chronic stress actually destroys brain cells and damages the hippocampus (the part of the brain that holds memory).[55]

The antidote is reducing stress, and we have already explored many tools for this including meditation, nutrition, and self-care. One promising piece of research has also shown that having an active social life with strong supportive relationships slows memory decline and improves emotional well-being.

Nutrition plays a crucial role in brain function, too. Eating real food such as whole grains, lots of fresh fruits and vegetables, healthy fats, and lean proteins has been shown to improve memory and brain function. Omega-3 fats are a well-researched ally in long-term brain development and health.[56] Green tea has also been shown to enhance memory and mental alertness.[57]

Another key to brain health is reducing inflammation. As inflammation around the nerves can cause damage to the brain, it is best to eat a healthy diet, reduce your contact with allergens, and make sure your gut is functioning well.

*5 tips for study time*[58]

1. **Eat before you learn.** Glucose improves memory. Take it in the form of a light snack, for a boost that will not drain your energy with a lot of digestive demands.

2. **Drink while you learn.** Hydration improves all body functions, including that of the brain.

3. **Use as many senses as you can.** Some people learn by reading, others by writing or hearing, while others need a combination of inputs. Be creative with this.

4. **Give the new material your 100% focus.** Learning requires your attention—and your intention.

5. **Repeat, and repeat again.** Rehearsing information as you learn it, either by retelling it to yourself or explaining it to someone else, helps you make an experiential connection to the material. Space this practice out at intervals during the study time, to build layers into your learning. This technique has been shown to work better than cramming.

## SPIRITUAL APPLICATION: *Times of Transition*

Autumn is the season of exhalation—the release. By exhaling and other forms of letting go, you are making space in yourself for something new, for something different, for the magic of transformation. You can support this energetically by having a good ol' material and emotional clear-out. Be fierce, and really let go of what you no longer need. Gift what you can to charity or friends. Give your home a smudge (see Global Apothecary, below) and make space to be empty and still, a blank page, full of potential.

Grief is one particularly appropriate emotion to tap during this time of gentle release. When you allow the stir of uncomfortable feelings to swirl around inside, you are able to bring them to the surface, to acknowledge them, thank them, and then release or integrate them as needed.

When you are able to feel grief deeply and honestly, you participate fully in the exhalation and release. This involvement allows you to receive the treasured gift of understanding that comes from grief—grasping what has real value in your life. This awareness can come with any transitional phase you approach; the change of seasons, loss of a job, moving to a new house, divorcing, the passing of a loved one, children entering puberty, and transitioning to a more independent life all contain some aspect of loss.

The power of the downward and introspective movement of autumnal energy allows you to let go of what is old, keep what is needed, and refine your awareness, offering you the gift of connecting again in a new and refreshed way.

## SOUL CHALLENGE: *Toning*

Western culture lacks grief rituals. It offers few ways to share the vast emotions of life transitions with your circle of family and friends. One way to express grief is through toning. Toning is the practice of making sounds that resonate with your emotional vibrations. Tapping into this vocal mystery, you will discover there is a sound that you can chant to balance each chakra. In times of grief and transition, the sound comes from your soul. Open your heart and tune in with your vocal cords. Allow whatever sounds to come out to speak your truths of grief.

## GLOBAL APOTHECARY: *Smudging*

Smudging is the practice of burning herbs, wood, or resins with the purpose of cleansing, clearing, and purifying a person or space. Some traditional tools include sage, rosemary, palo santo, dried bundles of other herbs, frankincense, or copal. Smudging has roots in many global healing traditions including Native American, Celtic, Asian, and Greek, to name a few. The purification happens through using the smoke in a focused, intentional way to cleanse negative energy and replenish positive, healing energy. Scientifically, the smoke from the herbs used in smudging has been shown to be antibacterial and antiviral.

When you smudge, it is important to show up mentally and energetically, and with focused intention. There is a job to be done, and it is not simply wafting a feather in smoke.

A few hospitals have rooms just for smudge ceremonies; however, some people have a negative reaction to smoke, and you are not always able to use smoke in places like hospitals or classrooms. Here are a few ways to achieve a similar cleansing result without burning.

- Clapping or ringing a bell in the corners and dark spaces of a room clears its energy.
- Drumming and dancing in a space raises the vibration.
- Auric Misters (see Chapter 10) lift the vibration with plant essences and essential oils.
- Laughter achieves pure beauty and light.
- Using flower essences (see Chapter 1) in your cleaning products changes the vibrational energy of your home.

## Conjuring and Crafting

### EASE ESSENCE

It is time to create another special essence for your medicine cupboard.

Tune into the feelings that arise during this time of transition. What do you and your family need most? Is it solace, balance, or ease?

Use an obsidian or aquamarine crystal—whichever resonates most strongly with the medicine you are making. You may choose to include a plant from nature. Trees are incredibly stabilizing, and usually very willing to help if asked.

Follow the "Making a Flower Essence" instructions in Chapter 1, keeping clearly focused on making an essence that will support you in times of transition.

## MEMORY AND CONCENTRATION OIL (FOR AN OIL-BURNER)

The intention of this blend is to calm and focus the mind.

- Oil-burner
- Tealight
- 3 drops basil essential oil
- 3 drops rosemary essential oil
- 3 drops frankincense essential oil
- 1 drop Ease Essence (above)
- Pure water

Add water to the basin of your oil-burner. Add essential oils and Ease Essence. Light the tealight and place it in the chamber under the basin.

Enjoy the aroma as it fills the room.

## CONCENTRATION BITES

These tasty treats are full of yummy and brain-boosting nutrients. They make the perfect studying, writing, and working snack.

- 1 cup almonds
- ½ cup walnuts

- 1 cup pitted medjool dates, chopped
- ¼ cup cacao powder
- 1 teaspoon pure vanilla extract
- 1 teaspoon rosewater
- Toppings—shredded coconut, cinnamon, sesame seeds, crushed pistachios, etc.
- 1 handful of determination
- 1 generous pinch of patience

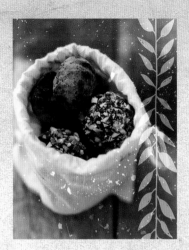

Grind almonds in a food processor. Add all the other ingredients, and blend until well combined and sticking together. Scrape out of the blender into a bowl, and roll into a ball. Roll the ball in your favorite superfood topping, and you are good to go!

Store in the refrigerator. These tasty treats also travel fine at room temperature for lunches.

## Pairings

- Plant Ally: Sage. Evidence has shown that sage extract can improve brain function, especially memory. This plant also dries well for homemade smudge bundles.
- Class: Sacred Loss is an in-depth exploration of grief and loss, held with the community of sisterhood in the Sacred Living Movement.
- Activity: Take up a new skill. Check out new offerings at your local community center and college to keep your brain agile with fresh new skills.

# Journal

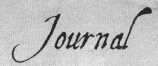

Twilight is a time of transition from one state of being to another. How do you flow through these changes? Use this space to dive deep into any grieving you may need to face at this time.

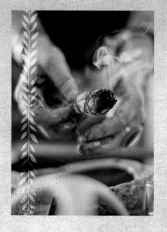

_____

_____

_____

_____

_____

_____

_____

_____

_____

_____

_____

_____

_____

_____

_____

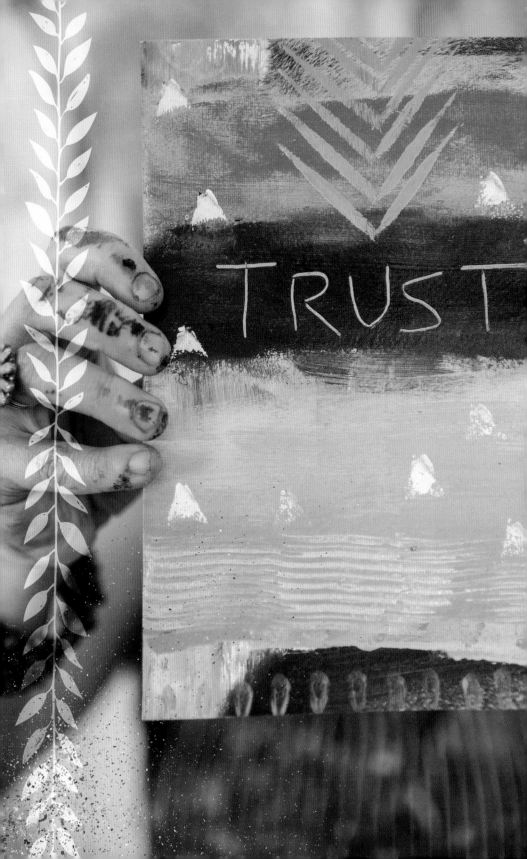

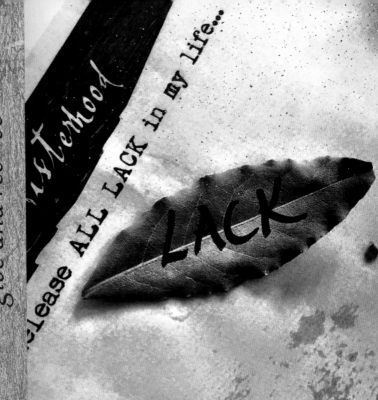

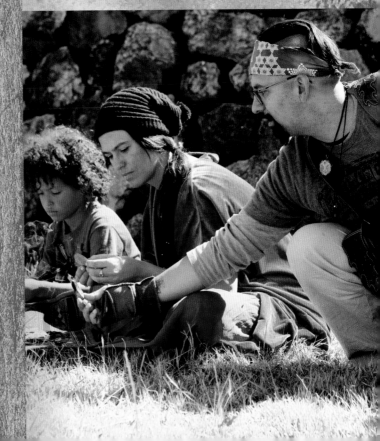

# abundance
*give and receive*

chapter 20

*Abundance is available to everyone who lives from a free and unconstrained mind. A maple tree full of orange, golden, and crimson leaves knows nothing of lack— only the seasons of change. There is no judgment surrounding the maple tree during barren winter, and likewise no celebration during the abundance of har- vest—only what is. An attitude of abundance is an understanding of gratitude for what you have in this moment in time.*

*If you live from an attitude of lack, you place a low-vibration quality on your feelings, so they can easily spiral into fear, anxiety, concern, and stress. The energy of giving and receiving go hand-in-hand and, with practice, can flow with the ease of a tree dropping its leaves as the wheel of the seasons turns.*

## FAMILY WELLNESS: *Living in Abundance*

You hold your loved ones with great care, and give with each breath to every member of your family. While this act of heart-generosity has huge payoffs, it can also deplete your internal resources. This is par- ticularly true if you live and breathe from a place of lack. How can you give your family the balanced energy they need to thrive, or find the energy you need to grow and prosper, when every ounce of you has "had it" and you are emotionally and physically spent? The answer is that you really can't—a dry well cannot offer up even a cup of water.

Living in abundance of spirit gives your family many ways to aspire to holistic wellness, and can give you the thrust of energy you need to accomplish everyday tasks with an elevated sense of self and purpose. This level of awareness directly affects the health of your family, as folks tend to get physically sick when they do not feel well on the inside.

### Hold family council once a week

Circle up as a family once a week, and do a check-in about how every- one is feeling and what is going on with each person emotionally and physically. Ask where they may be feeling depleted, and share your story as well. With this information, everyone can work toward a more regular balance and abundance of holistic health. End with lighting a candle of peace and abundance-of-wellness for your family for the next week, until you circle up again.

## SPIRITUAL APPLICATION: *Trust*

The universe conspires in every way to help us succeed and be healthy in life. When we live in trust that there is enough and will always be enough for all of us, we can release attachment to the "When I get this ... then that" syndrome, and just be grateful for our current life situation.

Trust is a biggie though—I get that! It can be easy for your manifestation guru to tell you to "just trust that everything in life will work out"; however, your personal stories and consciousness can make that a next-to-impossible task. When you are pushed, or when you really don't have enough money to pay the rent or buy food, is the time when "trust comes to shove." It's when trust gets wobbly, and our romance with it threatens to break up.

These are the moments when you need to send trust a dozen red roses, take her out for a gourmet meal, and write sappy love sonnets for her! Believing that life is a magical journey and that you are an integral part of the divine plan of destiny is a *must* step for bringing abundance of all kinds into your life. Your abundant life is waiting for you to just believe and say YES.

## SOUL CHALLENGE: *Non-Attachment*

Think of a personal possession that you love—something meaningful and special. Now think of someone in your life who would appreciate it as a gift. Mail it, or drop it off for them, letting them know what it means to you. Giving away something you love is a lesson in freeing yourself from attachment. This helps you stay in the flow of give-and-take.

## GLOBAL APOTHECARY: *Openness*

Abundance is free for those who seek it with pure intentions. Getting in right relationship with abundance means understanding your worth, understanding nonattachment, and living in gratitude. Give when you think you have nothing to give, understanding that the energetic flow of giving and receiving puts you in harmonious balance with abundance, and calls in all forms of it into your life. This process starts with returning to openness.

Openness is not something you can buy, but it's something everyone seeks. Therefore, this commodity becomes more valuable than anything you could buy or sell. Once you learn this rich and valuable life skill, not only are you holding onto one of the most valuable things in humanity, you are the keeper of energy.

When we come into the world, we are inherently open to absorb all that is around us. As time goes on, we get more and more closed, based on our particular life story. If you have gone far down that road, you need to come back home, to return to your birthright of openness. This is *crucial*.

You can be open to being loved, open to being wanted and seen as valuable, open to being heard and listened to, and open to the abundance of financial freedom. When you create freedom in your immediate world, you open yourself up to more and abundant freedoms in a way that stores the most valuable, untouchable commodity there is—your energy. Nobody can teach you this part. It's all just *you*.

## Conjuring and Crafting

### CALLING IN ABUNDANCE

Financial health and wellness are important to a well-balanced life. Taking time to unfold your relationship to finances and to cultivate financial freedom may also tell you a lot about other aspects in your life where you may be questioning your worth.

## BAY LEAF "LACK CHALLENGE"

Living in lack is staying in the place of fear—a place that keeps us tight instead of loose, stressed instead of free, closed down instead of open to opportunity. When you set your mind to something, you may just be able to manifest it if you approach it with clear, conscious intentions. When we live in lack, we focus on all that we *don't have rather than on what we do* have. So start by identifying whether you are a lack-focused or abundance-focused person in this moment.

To stop living in lack, try this ceremony. Take a bay leaf, write the word "lack" on it, and when you feel ready to expel lack from your life, *burn it!* You need to set your intention and mean it. Ask the bay leaf to speak to you through the fire. If the leaf crackles and burns brightly to the end of the leaf, then the outcome is positive; you really are ready to release your attachment to lack.

If the bay leaf just smolders or refuses to burn, then you know that somewhere inside of you fear is winning, and your focus on lack could be stopping you from fully trusting that your divine path will unfold and that you will always, and in all ways, be abundant. A good place to start is to examine your real beliefs about lack and prosperity. Do you believe there is enough for everyone in this world? Perhaps you assume you need to work very hard for a long time to be prosperous. Once you identify some of these underlying beliefs, you can begin working towards a more abundant state of mind.

## PROSPERITY OIL

Use this oil to anoint yourself everyday so that you will move through the world manifesting abundance and financial wellness in your life.

- Small glass bottle with a lid (the size of a baby-food jar)
- Enough carrier oil (almond or sesame are great) to fill half the jar
- 3 parts ginger essential oil
- 3 parts orange essential oil
- 4 parts pine essential oil
- 2 parts cinnamon essential oil
- 1 part chamomile essential oil
- 2 parts cedarwood essential oil
- 5 parts jasmine or lotus essential oil
- 2 parts rose essential oil
- A few loose dried rose petals
- 1 small citrine crystal
- 1 part real gold flakes

Fill half of the jar with your favorite carrier oil. Add as much of each essential oil that you are drawn to as you choose, using the above proportions as a guide. Add in the rose petals, citrine stone and gold flakes. Say a blessing over your oil, asking it to serve you in manifesting financial wellness in your life.

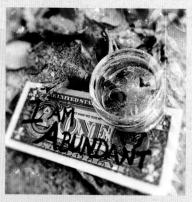

Remember to anoint your third-eye chakra every morning, as you dive into bringing forth what you want to manifest. You can also anoint a dollar bill and keep it in your wallet at all times.

# LAKSHMI MEDITATION

*Abundance is not something we acquire. It is something we tune into.*
—WAYNE DYER

We all need a little help from the gods and goddesses from time to time. Lakshmi is the Hindu goddess of prosperity, and she bestows her gold and treasures upon you when you live in harmony and balance. Take time to say a prayer to her, asking for her assistance affording you abundance in any form you need it.

- 1 picture of the Goddess Lakshmi (you can find one online and print it out)
- 1 candle to light in her honor
- Various coins

Put the picture of Lakshmi in your sacred space, and light a candle in her honor. Place the coins at the base of her feet (you may consider anointing them with Prosperity Oil, above). Ask her to gift you with abundance in the areas you need it most. Then thank her, and be sure to appreciate any offerings you receive in the days following.

## Pairings

- Online Class: Sacred Living Movement—Money Manifestation with Anni Daulter
- Crystal: Citrine is a yellowish crystal that calls on abundance to come into your life in all forms. You can wear a citrine necklace to have it with you at all times, or carry a stone in your bag; always have it close to you when working on calling in abundance.

# Journal

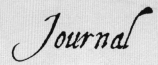

Be in gratitude for all that you have in this moment, and take the time to make a healthy list here of everything that you are grateful for:

_____

_____

_____

_____

_____

_____

_____

_____

_____

_____

_____

_____

_____

_____

_____

_____

_____

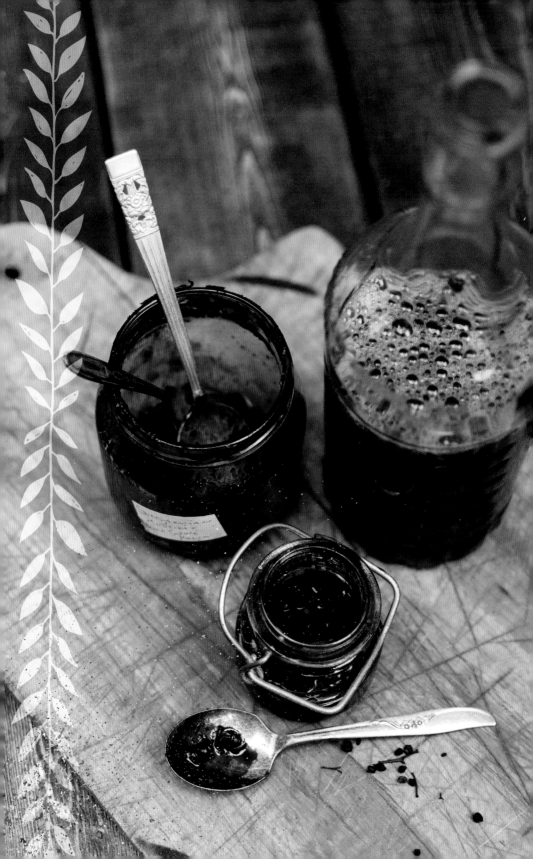

*autumn equinox*

*the soul harvest*

**chapter 21**

*Here you are, once again, in the time where the day and night weigh equally in the scales of the sky. You reflect on the soon-to-be-waning light, and feel the call of its slow quietude. Yet there is still time to inhale the sweet elixir of the bountiful harvest. There are feasts to be had, and autumn stores to be prepared.*

*Now is the time to pluck the last of the light and store it in your pocket for those dark, wet days ahead. Go ahead—reach up and grab it! The present is just for you. It is time to invoke your inner hearth goddess, and get to work. There is much to be done to gather in the gifts of this crisp season.*

## FAMILY WELLNESS: *A Foundation for Strong Immunity*

Immunity is the body's defense system, protecting it from harmful germs, parasites, and bacteria. To do this, the immune system needs to differentiate between healthy cells and the interlopers. This intricate system is a very complicated set of processes that science has only recently begun to understand. Your defenses include your skin, mucus membranes, digestive-tract bacteria, lymph nodes, and special cells including antibodies, lymphocytes, and phagocytes. Lymphocytes help the body recognize and destroy the invading agents of disease. Phagocytes primarily obliterate pathogens.[59]

Since the immune system has so many parts, it is hard for "boost the immune system" to be truly meaningful. The foundation of a robust immunity is a healthy lifestyle. The good news is that if you've put into place even a few of the tips in this book so far, you are already creating a foundation for strong immunity. Let's review some of these tips, and connect them with your vital energy.[60]

- **Eat a well-balanced diet.** Malnutrition, sadly, has been shown to prevent a strong immune response. If you are eating a varied, whole-grain- and plant-based diet, you are already getting an important range of micronutrients and vitamins. Nutrients such as zinc, selenium, and vitamins A, C, E, and D have all been shown to play a role in immune response, so by choosing "rainbow eating" you are providing the building blocks your body needs.

- **Break up with processed sugar.** Sugar has been shown to suppress the immune response. Eating less of it, especially when your body is already working hard to fight an illness, removes a harmful roadblock to your health.

- **Practice balanced hygiene.** Oversanitizing prevents developing immune systems from becoming robust. But balance day-to-day exposure with thoughtful hygiene practices; handwashing and covering your mouth when coughing or sneezing can prevent the spread of undesirable germs.

- **Stay hydrated.** Water flushes out toxins, helps produce lymph, supports digestion, and oxygenates the blood. These are all intrinsic parts of a well-functioning immune system.

- **Keep that body moving.** Rhythm and movement keep the lymph system flushing toxins through the body; they help the heart and lungs do their jobs, and reduce stress.

- **When in doubt, laugh.** Laughter helps reduce the stress hormone cortisol, and measurably increases antibodies.

## SPIRITUAL APPLICATION: *The Harvest of Your Soul*

Autumn Equinox has traditionally been celebrated as a harvest festival. Gathering in the bounty of your plantings, preserving sweet treasures for winter, sharing your abundance with your community and family—are all welcomed, loving moments of this season. It is a time of generosity and gratitude, and opening your home to others in need. From Autumn Equinox on, the long nights are becoming more evident, and the energy of the season is slowing down and spooling inward.

Take time in the pause between light and dark to assess your harvest. What plantings of your soul and health flourished? What failed to take root? What is it time to let go of? What is it time to preserve for the days ahead?

## SOUL CHALLENGE: *Blessing Tree*

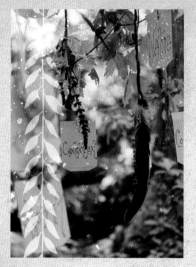

Honor your harvest by making a beautiful blessing tree. Use nature-friendly materials such as recycled paper, wool string, hemp twine, feathers, and crystals. Each person can write an example of their bounty on small cards, and use the wool/twine, feathers, and crystals to create a living blessing right in your garden. If you don't have access to a live tree that wants to be honored in this way, make one out of paper and hang it on your wall.

## GLOBAL APOTHECARY: *Throat Chakra*

The throat chakra, called *vishuddha,* is the gateway into the upper three spiritual chakras. This is the place where authentic heart truths are spoken. A balanced throat chakra allows you to listen with the ears of Spirit and speak your truth graciously, without the need to please or hurt others. The thyroid, mouth, jaw, neck, and throat areas are linked with the throat chakra. Chanting the mantra *"hum"* and wearing the color blue or lapis lazuli can help open and balance this chakra.[61]

## *Conjuring and Crafting*

These are our favorite immune-enhancing autumn recipes.

---

## GOLDEN IMMUNITY OINTMENT (BUBBLE BALM)

*This balm is not recommended for children under age two because of the essential oils.*

We also call this "Bubble Balm" because it wraps you in a protective bubble. We make lots of it as a gift ointment to share with aunties, uncles, grandparents, and friends!

- Two 3-ounce (travel-size) jars
- 4 ounces coconut oil
- 1 ounce beeswax
- 10 drops frankincense essential oil
- 10 drops clove essential oil
- 10 drops cinnamon leaf essential oil
- 3 drops yarrow flower essence

Melt coconut oil and beeswax in a double-boiler, or in a heatproof container set over a pan of water. As soon as they are melted, remove from heat and allow to cool slightly. Add essential oils and flower essence, and stir well. Pour into jars.

Dab a little around the nose, and rub into hands. Rub lovingly onto the soles of the feet at the first sign of a sniffle. You can also rub it onto the chest and back. This ointment is great for travel and the busy winter period.

**Note:** Cinnamon leaf essential oil is not recommended for people on anticoagulant medications, because it could interfere with blood clotting; substitute white pine or fir.

---

## ELDERBERRY AND ROSEHIP SYRUP

Elderberry (*Sambucus nigra*), also called common elder or black elder, has berries that are dark-purple, almost black. These contain organic pigments, tannin, amino acids, carotenoids, flavonoids, sugar, rutin, viburnic acid, vitamin A and B, and a large amount of vitamin C. Flavonoids, including quercetin, are believed to account for the therapeutic actions of the elderberry flowers and berries.[62] However, don't eat them raw, as they have a laxative effect if uncooked.

Humans have had a long and special relationship with the elder plant. We have used all of her gifts—bark, leaves, flowers and fruit—for making medicines, teas, jams, and drinks. It is believed that the fairies protect the elder; taking the wood without the right kind of ceremony and permission is considered very bad luck.

Rosehips are extremely high in vitamin C; together, this dynamic duo makes a powerful immune-enhancing tonic for the fall.

- Two sterile 16-ounce jars or bottles
- Strainer or sieve
- Cheesecloth
- 8 ounces fresh rose hips (*Rosa canina*) or 4 ounces dried rosehips
- 8 ounces fresh elderberries (*Sambucus nigra*) or 4 ounces dried elderberries
- 2 quarts pure water
- 5 clove buds
- 1 cinnamon stick
- 13 ounces organic sugar (can also use coconut sugar or maple syrup)

If using fresh rose hips, clean and remove the stalks, and chop them. Using a food processor is easiest. If using fresh elderberries, remove berries from the stems with a fork, and mash them a little.

Bring to boil 1½ quarts of the water in a large pot. Add berries, cloves, and cinnamon stick, and bring back to boil. Remove from heat and allow to steep for 20 minutes. Pour into a sieve lined with cheesecloth and placed over a bowl, and allow liquid to drip through. Set aside the strained liquid and add fruit pulp back to pan with the remaining pint of water. Bring back to a boil, then turn off heat and let steep for 20 minutes once more. Drain through the cheesecloth-lined sieve as before.

In a pan, mix together both batches of strained juice and sugar. Bring to a boil and simmer for a few minutes, until the sugar is dissolved and the consistency is syrupy. Pour syrup into jars or bottles while hot, and seal them following manufacturer's directions for your containers.

To serve, we like to put 2–3 Tablespoons of syrup in a mug with 3–4 cloves and a squeeze of lemon juice, then top with hot water—and enjoy.

## Pairings

· Tool: Miron violet glass bottles—these beautiful glass jars and bottles are worth the investment for your favorite recipes, as the color of the glass offers optimal protection against the aging processes that occur from exposure to light.

· Act of Service: Share the bounty of your harvest with others—donate to, or volunteer at, your local food bank.

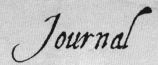

# Journal

Take time this week to check in with
your wellness practices for the coming
season. Now is a good time to do a new
basic check-in from the Family Wellness
section of Chapter 1: How are you doing?
What is flourishing? What needs a little
support?

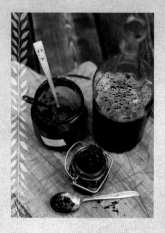

_____

_____

_____

_____

_____

_____

_____

_____

_____

_____

_____

_____

_____

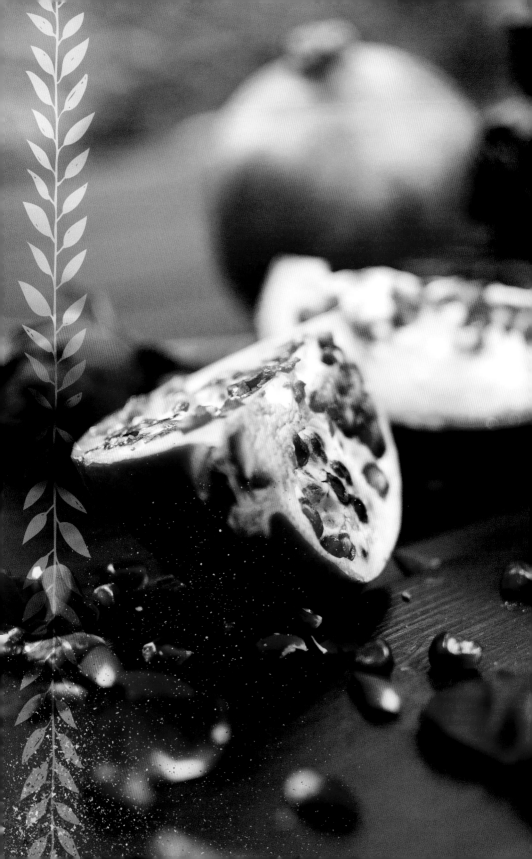

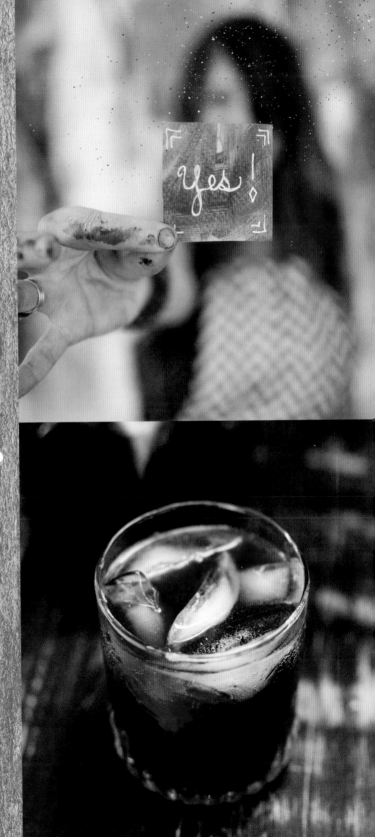

# the fruit

## ripening with grace

chapter 22

There are few things more beautiful or tempting than a luscious fruit allowed to linger and ripen at its own pace on the tree. The process of time ages it to perfection, and the nourishment from light and water infuses the fruit with tantalizing juiciness. In the natural cycle of the plant, blossom follows bud, and fruit forms from the flower. The beauty of the fruit is in its maturity.

As you grow through life and approach your own threshold into adulthood, revel in the awareness that these ripe years offer abundant opportunities to express your full creativity, root deeply into community, and flourish into your full potential.

## FAMILY WELLNESS: *Antioxidants*

Antioxidants protect your cells and DNA from free-radical damage. Free radicals are caused by oxidation, which is a normal, essential process in the daily life of the cell. When oxygen breaks down as cells use it, the leftover parts of oxygen and other atoms can become free radicals. These cellular byproducts can cause issues like cell mutations, which in turn lead to disease and premature aging.

Antioxidants counter these effects by bonding to the leftover molecules and sweeping them out of the body. They also support your immune system and overall vitality. The main antioxidants in our diet are vitamins A, C, and E, plus the minerals selenium and zinc. Recent studies suggest that supplementation is not necessary; you can get what you need through a healthy diet.[63]

A few sources of food high in antioxidants are blueberries, pomegranates, grapes, dark chocolate, pecans, elderberries, rosehips, cilantro, and artichokes.[64]

## SPIRITUAL APPLICATION: *Self-Care—Careful Nurturing*

How do you love yourself? This is important because, if you cannot see the beauty and wonder of your own heart, how can others? If you cannot respect your health on all levels—physical, mental, emotional, and spiritual—how will your children know that these parts of themselves have value? This sense of worth extends outward, to your partner and to your community.

Self-care is the ultimate act of service to yourself and the larger world. It is not a luxury, a treat, a self-indulgence, or a way to "spoil yourself." That kind of language about self-care depreciates the value of what is essential, impeccable, and loving. Being able to care for yourself directly benefits you and your whole family. By caring for yourself, you consciously create a strong center, which allows you to give from a place of stability and confidence.

*And here is another important fact:* You can't truly give from a place of emptiness or lack—which only further depletes your resources and energy. Fill yourself up with an abundance of care, and you will have personal resources to share.

## SOUL CHALLENGE: *Self-Care Vow*

Take a moment to make a sacred vow to yourself about how you will care for YOU. Anything you do that fills your heart and spirit, that honors the wonder of your consciousness and your body, is impeccable self-care.

This doesn't have to be expensive or complicated. Mindful breathing, walking in nature, or reading something that reminds you of love are just a few ways to fill your cup. Dancing, singing, drumming, playing, and celebrating the simple wonder of our being are even more ways to elevate this vow to sacredness. Embracing your "Holy NO!" and having clear boundaries, taking time for yourself with a long bath or shower, anointing yourself with scented oils, flower essences, and crystals, and living in the Beauty Way (the practice of noticing fine details, cultivating beauty in every aspect of life, and touching every soul you meet with your own personal brand of beauty medicine) through your words and actions are even more ways to live out your vow.

All of these small acts are gifts to yourself, to make your heartspace more beautiful and abundant. The more you put in, the more there is to flow out, allowing you to sprinkle everyone one around you with your abundant love-dust.

## GLOBAL APOTHECARY: *Pomegranates*

There are few fruits more lush and ripe with potential than a pomegranate. Ancient cultures associated this fruit with women's most sacred treasure, the secret jewels of the womb. They have long been considered aphrodisiacs, and used in global medicine traditions to improve fertility for both men and women.

This plant gives on all levels. As a flower essence, pomegranate is a woman's friend, balancing the sacral chakra and overall energy flow. The pomegranate flower herself is deeply feminine, flirty, and sensual. This energy teaches us how to touch those places in ourselves and awaken them in powerful ways.

As food, pomegranates are high in antioxidants, folic acid, and vital nutrients. They can be added to teas or smoothies, juiced, or eaten raw or cooked.

## *Conjuring and Crafting*

Welcome the sensual and divine essence of pomegranate into your life with these recipes.

### POMEGRANATE SUGAR SCRUB

This lush and vibrant scrub brings a glow to your skin.

- 1 large, airtight jar
- 4 cups granulated sugar
- ½ cup coconut oil
- ¼ cup infused orange oil
- ¼ cup fresh pomegranate juice

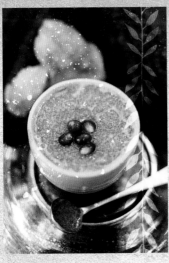

- 21 drops of benzoin essential oil
- Zest of 1 organic orange
- 3 drops pomegranate flower essence

Put the sugar and coconut oil into a large bowl. Mix until well combined. If the coconut oil is too hard, warm it gently in a double-boiler, or in a heat-proof container on a pan of hot water, until just softened. Add the pomegranate juice, essential oil, and flower essence, and combine until mixed well and you like the texture.

Spoon scrub into your jar. Decorate a label for it, and indulge in impeccable self-care.

## SPICED POMEGRANATE SYRUP

This makes a great base for party punch, and a topping for ice cream and desserts.

- 1 32-ounce bottle of organic 100% pomegranate juice (no added sugar)
- ¼ cup organic sugar—either raw, organic cane sugar or coconut sugar
- ¼ cup maple syrup
- 1 Tablespoon molasses
- 1 Tablespoon fresh lemon or orange juice
- 1 cinnamon stick
- 3 drops pomegranate flower essence

Add all the ingredients to a saucepan except the flower essence, and bring to a boil over medium heat. Once boiling, turn heat down to a steady simmer. Simmer until reduced by at least half, and the consistency is thick and syrupy. Remove from heat and add flower essence. Allow to cool completely, and store in fridge.

Add a couple of Tablespoons to a glass and top with sparkling water. Or add it to your best party-punch recipe. This syrup is also delicious on pancakes.

---

## POMEGRANATE GLOW SERUM

A nourishing blend for facial care.

- $1\frac{1}{2}$-ounce dropper bottle
- 2 teaspoons pomegranate oil
- 2 Tablespoons rosehip oil
- 2 teaspoons rose oil
- $\frac{1}{2}$ teaspoon vitamin E
- 3 drops myrrh essential oil
- 3 drops geranium essential oil
- 3 drops neroli essential oil
- 3 drops white lotus flower essence

Mix all the ingredients together in a small measuring jug. Pour into bottle.

Apply by putting a few drops into your hand and massaging them into your face.

*Pairings*

- Tool: Monthly self-care box subscription. These little care packages arrive with new treats each month. We love Honey and Sage in the USA, and Rainbow Soul in the UK. Created by women, for women.
- Activity: Spa day or pamper night with your friends. Fill your cups together with the light of community and the glow of self-care.

# *Journal*

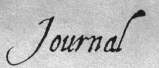

Create a list of ways to fill your cup. What is your self-care vow?

_____

_____

_____

_____

_____

_____

_____

_____

_____

_____

_____

_____

_____

_____

_____

_____

_____

_____

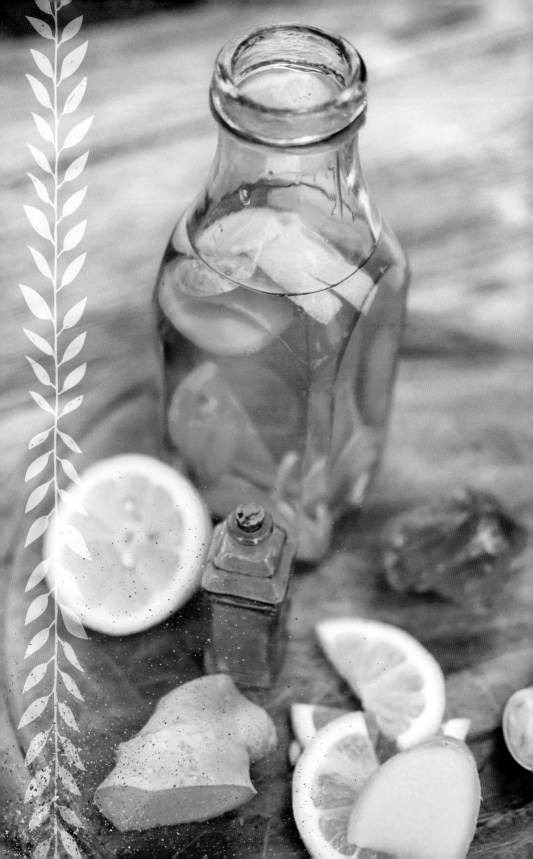

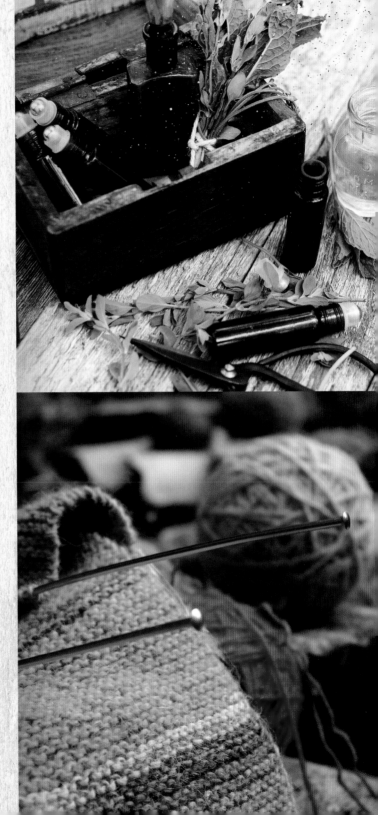

*nurture*

actions speak louder than words

chapter 23

*A soft touch, a gentle whisper, a loving glance, a home-cooked meal, a strong hug, a gentle kiss, or cuddling in a warm knitted blanket can all be forms of nurturing. While it comes in many forms, the outcome is always and in all ways dependable— it waters the tender soul and feeds the growing mind. Nurturing is a heartfelt act of service to yourself and to those you love; it replenishes the deep reservoirs of love and connection like nothing else. When you use these superpowers to help someone else, you elevate humanity and raise your vibration to living in your highest self.*

## FAMILY WELLNESS: *Stress*

One of the most common causes of disease in today's world is stress. While the causes of stress change from person to person, the resulting physical effects in the body are consistent. One of these is the activation of the hormone cortisol. Called "the stress hormone," cortisol is produced by your adrenal glands and influences many functions of the body. Here are just a few of the physical functions affected by cortisol:

- Blood-sugar (glucose) levels
- Fat, protein, and carbohydrate metabolism
- Immune responses
- Anti-inflammatory actions
- Blood pressure
- Heart and blood-vessel tone and contraction
- Central nervous system activation

In an ordinary stress situation, the adrenals secrete more cortisol. Then, ideally, once the stress has passed, bodily functions and cortisol levels drop back to normal. The reality is, in our present stress-filled culture, the stress response is activated so often that the body does not always rebalance.[65, 66]

### Favorite stress-busters

- **Feed your adrenals.** B vitamins help your body cope with the effects of stress, and more vitamin C is in your adrenals than anywhere else in the body. Salt is another resource used up by stress, so replenish your supplies with a balanced sea salt, or a tasty broth.

· **Teach your body what a relaxed state feels like.** For some people, meditation or mindfulness can achieve this. For others, bodywork such as shiatsu, massage, or reflexology can help. Once your body remembers how to relax, you can use your mind to reach this state on your own.

· **Deal with stress triggers!** If your stress is overwork, school, or trauma exposure, seek support structures to relieve these potential pressures. Asking for help, slowing down, and acknowledging hard emotional triggers are all excellent beginning steps to relieving these stressors. Further assists could include tools such as hypnotherapy, or body movement such as yoga or belly dancing.

· **Be generous with yourself.** Create space and time to do what you love. Maybe you would like to go for a walk in nature, meditate, swim, go shopping, or catch a funny movie. Taking care of yourself in this way expands your ability to give to others.

· **Spend time in nature.** It has been scientifically proven that even just fifteen minutes in nature reduces stress levels. So turn off the screens and enjoy some sun, sea, and land.

## SPIRITUAL APPLICATION: *Beyond Survival*

In the whirlwind of daily life, it is easy to lose sight of what is most precious. Sometimes survival takes all your energy—working, getting meals on the table, and keeping a roof over everyone's head. These tasks are important, but living in physical and spiritual "survival mode" is not sustainable. Nurturing your own soul is just as important as taking care of day-to-day tasks.

Small gestures of beauty and meaning are the antidote to the white noise of survival mode. Sipping the deep drink of your life by actually smelling the roses, savoring the scent and flavor of your favorite cup of tea, or giving your beloved a lover's glance are all practices that can elevate the mundane to Sacred Living.

## SOUL CHALLENGE: *Single-Tasking*

Focus on the present moment with mindful intention by doing one thing at a time. Normally, you may simultaneously look out the window, make a cup of tea, and do the laundry. Try slowing down that process, and unfold each part of it as a separate present moment. Feel it with all of your senses.

## GLOBAL APOTHECARY: *Acupressure*

Acupressure is the ancient art of applying pressure to specific healing points on the body with the fingers. It is part of Asian medicine traditions, and uses the same points as acupuncture. Some benefits of acupressure include the release of muscular tension, support of the blood circulation, and balancing of body energy.

### *A sweet acupressure point to try*

A lovely way to calm stress is to connect the acupressure point called Kidney 1, or "Gushing Spring," located on the sole of the foot between the second and third metatarsal bones, approximately one-third of the distance between the base of the second toe and the heel, in a depression formed when the foot is plantar (downward)-flexed. Basically, this point is in the middle of the sole of your foot.[67]

    Sit comfortably and rest your ankle on your knee, so you that can reach your foot. Gently press the soft point in the center of your sole. Feel the energy move through your body, descending from your head to your lower back and spooling down into your legs. Allow your breath to flow along with the energy, and relax and be still. This moment is a gift for you.

# Conjuring and Crafting

Nurture yourself and your loved ones with these gentle recipes, intended to soothe and restore the body and mind.

## TUMMY TEA

This tea is a delicious and calming blend for sore tummies and spirits. Make extra, and gift some to a friend for a rainy day.

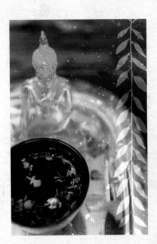

- ½ cup dried lemon balm
- ¼ cup dried chamomile
- ¼ cup fennel seeds
- ¼ cup dried ginger root
- ¼ cup dried catnip

Simply mix the herbs together and keep in a sealed jar. When needed, brew I heaping Tablespoon in a teapot for about 10 minutes. Strain and serve. Sweeten with honey if you like.

## GINGER AND APPLE CIDER VINEGAR TONIC

Ginger and apple cider vinegar are both wonderful for settling a rumbly tummy. The vinegar's ability to tame unfriendly intestinal bacteria and yeast provides the added benefit of promoting overall gut-flora balance. You can take this tonic everyday in the morning.

- 10 ounces pure water
- 3 slices ginger root
- 1–2 teaspoons raw apple cider vinegar
- Squeeze of lemon juice
- Honey, to taste

Bring water and ginger to a boil in a pan. Turn off heat and allow to cool to drinking temperature. Strain out the ginger, add the rest of the ingredients, and mix well.

Enjoy each morning, or anytime you have mild tummy trouble.

---

## SOOTHING HEADACHE ROLLERBALL

*Note: This remedy is not recommended for children.*

This travel-size blend is a trusted friend when tension strikes.

- ⅓-ounce (10-ml.) rollerball tube with ball and lid
- Plastic pipette
- Small bowl or measuring jug
- ¼ ounce of carrier oil such as rose oil or almond oil
- 10 drops peppermint essential oil
- 10 drops marjoram essential oil
- 10 drops lavender essential oil
- 10 drops bergamot essential oil
- 3 drops iris or self-heal flower essence

Mix together carrier oil, essential oils, and flower essence in the bowl or measuring jug. Use the plastic pipette to transfer the oil mixture into the rollerball.

Roll on back of neck, pulse points, and temples (around the hairline—avoid contact with eyes). You can also rub it into your hands, cup hands near your nose, and inhale.

## Pairings

- Music: *Everyone Deserves Music* by Michael Franti and Spearhead—a relaxing and uplifting album.
- Book: *Acupressure's Potent Points: A Guide to Self-Care for Common Ailments* by Michael Reed Gach. A classic compendium of points for the layperson to practice at home.

# Journal

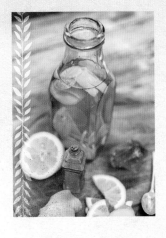

What is your favorite kind of nurturing
to give? What is your favorite kind of
nurturing to receive? How do you nurture
these love languages in your family?

_____

_____

_____

_____

_____

_____

_____

_____

_____

_____

_____

_____

_____

_____

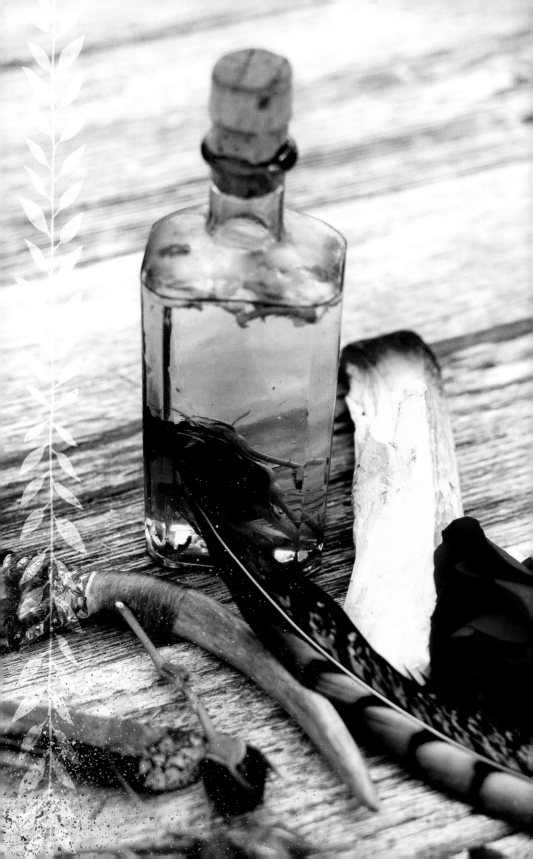

# rite

*honoring the ceremonial flow*

chapter 24

*It is your birthright to celebrate the milestones of humanity—birth, puberty, marriage, death, transition, triumph, failure, menopause, and liberation. Ritual, ceremony, and rites of passage may seem to be mysterious old-world teachings in today's modern society, but the practice of ceremony is hardwired into your soul. If you allow space for it to unfold, your guardians, ancestors, and spirit guides will share and gift you with an understanding of these ancient rites, so that they can live on in humanity. All you have to do is hear the call and respond with a whole-body YES, and the information will be passed down to you.*

*Allow the song of your heart to guide you. There is no occasion too small, no ceremony too mundane. Honor the seasons of your life with words, songs, tears, dance, remembrance, and purpose.*

## FAMILY WELLNESS: *Rites of Passage*

At its essential core, a rite of passage is a ceremony that honors life transitions. For a woman, the most fundamental of these transitions are birth, puberty, and menopause. It has been shown that how young women experience their first menses impacts the rest of their life.[68] While it may not have been studied yet, we would say this is true for young men as well. How will young people know their body has value, their spirit has merit, and their community sees those things, unless they are marked and celebrated? The same is true for elders in our lives as well. Marking these changing roles, and honoring the value of wisdom gained, promotes long-term emotional and community well-being.

A rite of passage can be a simple personal ceremony or a larger, more organized event. The key is your attitude and intention. Walking over a bridge to symbolize leaving the old behind and moving to the new is one kind of ceremony. Taking a remnant of the old life and replacing it with a new tool or symbol of a new skill is another method. The most important aspect is being witnessed, seen, and recognized for the change. Wisdom-keepers from cultures all around the world have protected this knowledge for us. With great respect and gratitude, it is time to take up the duty of creating ceremony, to authentically witness your journey and the path of your loved ones.

## SPIRITUAL APPLICATION: *Ceremony 101*

The bones of creating ceremony are very simple. Set your intention, invoke Spirit, be witnessed in your intention, and then close with gratitude. The many nuances of location, size, season, and meaning are completely variable and can be tied to any cultural or religious system you have chosen. What matters is that you select aspects that are authentic to you and the people you are sharing ceremony with. Rituals are the most potent when they are held in a language and with symbols that participants connect with.

### A basic outline for personal ceremonies

You can adapt this to make it resonate within you.

1. **Set your clear intention by stating what the ceremony is about.** For example: This ceremony is to honor first menses, say goodbye to an old job, or celebrate a college graduation.

2. **Select your ceremonial items.** Gather a candle, and two items that represent the old life and the new, such as objects representing old and new activities.

3. **Choose your space for the ceremony, and clean it.** It could be an altar in your home, a room, or somewhere in nature. You can prepare the area with smudging using white sage or palo santo, or with the Cleaning Powder from Chapter 1, an Auric Mister (Chapter 10), and/or drumming.

4. **Clean yourself.** Prepare for the ceremony by bathing, perhaps with a Cleansing Plant Bundle (Chapter 6) or an Auric Mister (Chapter 10).

5. **When you are ready, open the ceremony.** Begin by lighting the candle and inviting in your benevolent spirit guides, higher self,

guardian angels, or any other spiritual helpers. Ask them to protect and witness you in this work.

6. **Hold the item that represents your old life.** Say: I see this tool, and I have integrated the lessons shared with me during this time. I set this tool aside with gratitude and honoring.

7. **Pick up the item that represents your new life.** Say: I accept this tool. I open to the gifts that this tool and this new life path may bring.

8. **Hold the tool to your heart.** Close your eyes and open to any thoughts, images, memories, or feelings that arise as you hold the tool.

9. **Be in gratitude.** When you are ready, thank your guides.

10. **Close the ceremony** by snuffing out the candle.

11. **Finish this ritual** by gifting the object that represented your old life to someone else in that stage of life.

## SOUL CHALLENGE: *Ceremony*

Put this work into practice. The more ceremonies you hold, the more you will feel comfortable with them. Design a small ceremony to mark a passage in your life or someone you love.

## GLOBAL APOTHECARY: *Drumming*

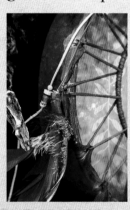

Drums are used by almost every culture in ceremony, music, ritual, and healing. Binaural rhythm has been known to help induce trance states for journeys into other worlds. In some traditions, drums have been used to call spirits, heal the wounded, and inspire people in times of despair. More recently, drumming therapy has been introduced to help people recover from addiction. A sense of rhythm is so innate to our core that even fetuses have been shown to have it. There is a timeless knowing that connects people with the beat of the drum and the rhythmic beat of the heart.

## Conjuring and Crafting

---

### TRANSITION MISTER

This auric mister can be used to prepare ceremonial space and honor times of transition.

- Small measuring cup
- 2-ounce mister bottle
- 10 drops sandalwood
- 10 drops cypress essential oil
- 10 drops rose essential oil
- 3 drops yarrow flower essence
- 1 teaspoon vanilla extract
- 1½ ounces pure water

Mix essential oils, flower essence, and vanilla extract together in measuring cup. Top with pure water and mix well. Pour into mister bottle, close lid, and give a good shake.

Mist around the ceremonial space and your auric field as needed.

---

### WARRIOR ANOINTING OIL

This is a woody and rooted oil to use in ceremonies that honor the Spiritual Warrior.

- Small measuring cup
- 2-ounce bottle

- 2 ounces almond oil

- 5 red rose petals

- 15 drops palo santo essential oil

- 15 drops sweet orange essential oil

- 10 drops sage essential oil

- 3 drops oak essence

Mix the oils and flower essence together in measuring cup. Pour into bottle.

Pour a small amount onto your finger, and anoint the center of the forehead, palms of hands, and soles of feet.

## Pairings

- Book: *Creating Ceremony* by Glennie Kindred and Lu Garner—a timeless reference for creating ritual.

- Class: Priestess Path with Nikiah Seeds at the Red Moon Mystery School. Take the work of ceremony and archetypes deeper, and step onto the life-changing path of the mystery school.

- Oracle Deck: *Sacred Rebels Oracle* by Alana Fairchild and Autumn Skye Morrison—a fascinating and beautifully illustrated oracle deck.

# *Journal*

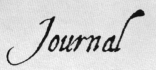

Use this space to dream up delicious
rituals:

_____

_____

_____

_____

_____

_____

_____

_____

_____

_____

_____

_____

_____

_____

_____

_____

_____

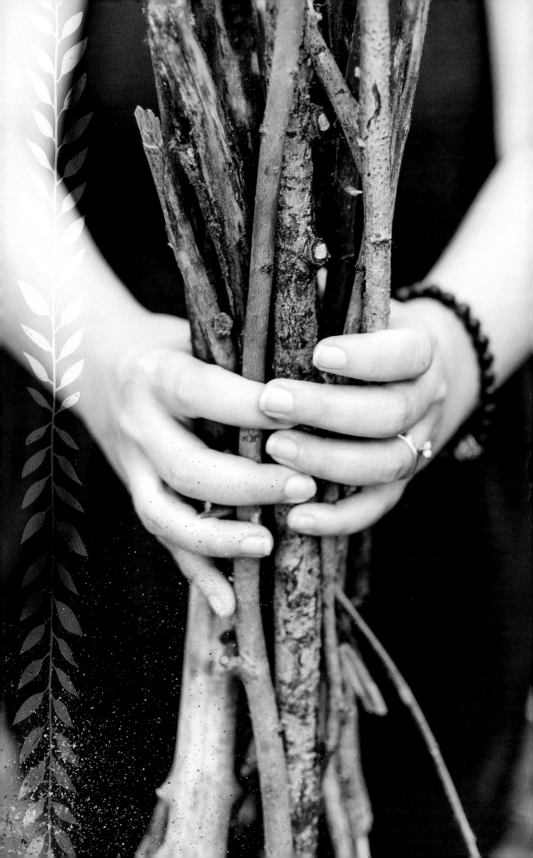

# gather

## the path of kinship

chapter 25

*As the season begins to darken, the crisp, chilled air beckons you to collect your resources for the long winter ahead. Gathering means calling back your energy from scattered projects and places, preserving your harvest, and sharing your abundance. Enfold yourself in the warmth of community and the strength of gratitude. This fostering of kinship keeps the fires of the spirit fueled and burning.*

## FAMILY WELLNESS: *Cold-Busters*

Even with the best of care, sometimes a cold still manages to get the better of you. Every body needs a good physical and emotional clear-out every now and again, and colds seem to serve this purpose.

While most colds just need to run their course, you can support your body by managing the symptoms. Here are some of our tried-and-tested favorites:

- **Hot drinks** provide hydration to flush out toxins and soothe sensitive mucus membranes in the throat.

- **Elevate your head** with pillows to support sinus drainage.

- **Warmth**: When your sinuses are inflamed, a warm compress on the face can make all the difference in the world. Take a washcloth and run it under warm water. Add a few drops of lavender flower essence, and place it over your eyes and across the top of your nose, leaving space to breathe. Press from the inside corner of your eyes out to your ears; this is the direction the lymph drains on your face. The heat from the compress helps open up the nasal passages; the lavender calms, and the massage helps to drain your swollen tissues.

- **Steam inhalations**: Add a few drops of essential oil and flower essence to a bowl of freshly boiled water. Place a towel over your head to make a little tent as you lean over the bowl. Breathe in the steam, and relax.

- **Rest, laughter, nourishment**: These are the basics. Rest gives your body time to do the work of healing, and laughter and nourishment support your immune system.

# SPIRITUAL APPLICATION: *Preserving and Sharing*

All of the work, energy, and effort you have put in over the changing of the seasons has laid the foundation for health and well-being. To gather your own harvest is to pull your resources inward and preserve your bounty, to properly prepare for the winter months of contemplation and good-quality home time. When you have an abundant crop of success, be it physical, energetic, or spiritual, you are able to live in the world more generously.

One divine aspect of a harvest well gathered is the sharing of the bounty in community. Not everyone has the same harvest to gather—some people grow carrots, others grow calm, and still others grow inspiration. Living connected to community is another resource to bulk up the pantry of the spirit. Cultivating and sharing in your community is the natural next step of a heart that is in balance.

# SOUL CHALLENGE: *Clean Energy*

This is an important process for taking care of your spirit. Calling your energy back to yourself gives you balanced integrity. It is a clean spiritual practice, and wonderful for boosting internal energy storage. For children, especially sensitive little ones, standing strong in their own energy can be very helpful. The process of calling back your energy requires a little practice, patience, and an open mind to get it rolling. This practice can be an elaborate one done in ceremony, or it can be quick and easy, done anywhere, anytime.

*Just say it! Calling back your energy*

**Caution:** This is not for pregnant mamas, or mamas with babies—please use the variation at the end of this method.

Use your mind to set the stage, and employ clear speech that you can speak with your whole heart, and mean it!

"I lovingly call back all of my energy from the past, present, and future. I call back my energy from wherever I left it, and from whomever it has attached to, intentionally or unintentionally. With love and compassion, I call back my energy to myself, to my center, to my source. I am whole. I am complete. I AM _____ *(say your whole name here)*!"

"I lovingly release any energy that does not belong to me. With gentle compassion, I send all energy that is not mine to its home—find your own center and your own place. I am whole. I am complete. I AM _____ *(say your whole name here)*!"

*For babies:* Because babies attach so completely to parents energetically (especially mothers or their primary caregivers), you want to be careful not to accidentally dump energy onto a new being. To help babies embody their Spirit and to clear their aura, gently rub the soles of their feet. Look into their eyes and say their name clearly three times, like a command: "*(Baby's full name),* this is your body. You are here now. This is your body."

*For pregnant mamas:* Use these words: "I am in balance with myself. I am in balance with the universe. I release all that does not serve me or my growing baby. I call back all of my energy with love, here and now."

## GLOBAL APOTHECARY: *Neti Pot*

A neti pot is a small pot from the Ayurvedic tradition. It is filled with salt and warm distilled or sterilized water. The saltwater is poured into the nose to rinse out congested nasal and sinus passages. It has been known to help with allergies, sinus problems, facial pain, and pressure. It is very important to use sterilized or distilled water because tap water could introduce infection. To learn more about using a neti pot, check out our Sacred Ayurveda program.

# *Conjuring and Crafting*

---

## COMMUNITY STONE SOUP

"Stone Soup" is an old fable that revolves around the story of bringing community together with a simple, humble soup made of nothing but water and a stone—*plus* a small food contribution from each person in the community. The stone at the bottom represents the whole of the community. This is a wonderful way to celebrate your gathered harvest of the year. Share your abundance with those you love.

- I cleaned river stone
- 4 cups water
- 6 cups chicken or vegetable broth
- I Tablespoon butter
- I yellow onion, chopped
- 3 garlic cloves, chopped
- 3 celery ribs, chopped
- 2 zucchini, chopped
- 3 carrots, chopped
- 3 red potatoes, chopped
- 2 Tablespoons soy sauce
- I teaspoon sea salt
- I teaspoon black pepper
- 2 teaspoons garlic salt

Start with a large pot and your river stone. Clean your river stone well, bless the stone with a prayer of deep nourishment, and place it at the bottom of the pot. Add the 4 cups of water and 6 cups of stock to the pot, and start heating it up to a simmer while everything else is being prepared.

Because this is a community effort, make sure each guest has a hand in preparing the soup and adding energy to the pot. Allow each guest to chop the vegetables. Feel free to add more vegetables as you desire. While the guests are happily chopping away, grab another large pot and melt your butter. Sauté the onions and garlic and, when they are lightly browned, add in the celery ribs, zucchini, carrots, and potatoes. Season all of that with the soy sauce, salt, pepper, and garlic salt. This process should take 6–8 minutes.

Add the vegetable sauté to the simmering pot of stock, and let all the flavors meld together. Continue to add salt and pepper to taste. You may want a little more soy sauce for extra flavor. Heat all of this to boiling; then turn down the heat and let simmer, to get final touches of flavor in the soup.

Serve warm to your community. You may want to offer Parmesan cheese as a topping. Before everyone eats, ask each person to turn to the person next to them and say, "May you never hunger." Then all enjoy the meal together.

---

## ONION AND HONEY POULTICE

*Note: Not recommended for children under two years old.*

Poultices are packets of herbs placed over an injury or affected area to support healing. Keeping cheesecloth in your medicine cupboard makes this an easy remedy to try. This poultice is a practical folk remedy that works very well for coughs and colds that just won't quit.

- Cheesecloth
- Hot-water bottle
- Towel
- 2 onions, chopped
- 3 Tablespoons olive oil

- 3 Tablespoons honey
- 3 Tablespoons flour
- 3 drops yarrow or grass of Parnassus flower essence

Heat the onions gently in the oil, until just translucent and fragrant. Remove from heat and add honey, mixing well. Then add in the flour until a sort of chunky onion paste is made. Spread this over half of the cheesecloth, then fold over the other half to cover the paste.

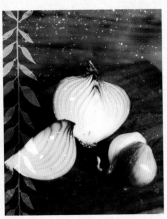

Make sure the contents are not too hot before placing on anyone! Place on upper back or upper chest—whichever is more comfortable. Do not cover the heart area. Place hot-water bottle on top, taking care to make sure it is not too hot. This should not be painful; it should be pleasantly warming. Cover everything with a towel, and rest for 15–20 minutes. Less is more for young or sensitive people. If doing this with children, make a lovely nesting place for them to rest with cozy pillows, books to read, or even a favorite movie; 5–20 minutes can be a long time for a child not to move. Can be repeated every 4–6 hours.

## COMPRESSES

Compresses, defined as a flat pad of material pressed onto the body, have been used by many traditions around the world. They are an easy home remedy, and a staple of any medicine cupboard.

**Hot Compresses** include hot-water bottles, heating pads, and warm, damp towels. Take care to check the temperature, and protect the skin from direct contact with the heat. Use heat to:

- Increase circulation
- Reduce stiffness and cramps
- Relax the body

**Cold Compresses** include ice packs, cold damp towels, or even bags of frozen peas. Take care to wrap the cold item in a damp towel to protect the skin from ice burns. Use cold to:

- Numb an injured area
- Reduce swelling and inflammation
- Slow down bleeding

## *Pairings*

- Website: www.bearmedicineherbals.com—Kiva Rose provides lovely, well-researched, in-depth information on herbal medicine practices including poultices.

- Nature Ally: Manuka honey from New Zealand—a potent antibacterial honey with healing properties. To be considered powerful enough to be therapeutic, manuka honey needs a minimum rating of 10 UMF (on the grading scale for manuka honey).

- Kid's Book: *Stone Soup* by Jon J. Muth. A tale of kindly monks who share a life lesson with a downhearted village, where ultimately all come together to nourish each other.

# *Journal*

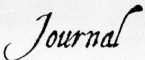

Practice the above Soul Challenge ("Clean Energy") every day for a week. How do you feel after this work?

_____

_____

_____

_____

_____

_____

_____

_____

_____

_____

_____

_____

_____

_____

_____

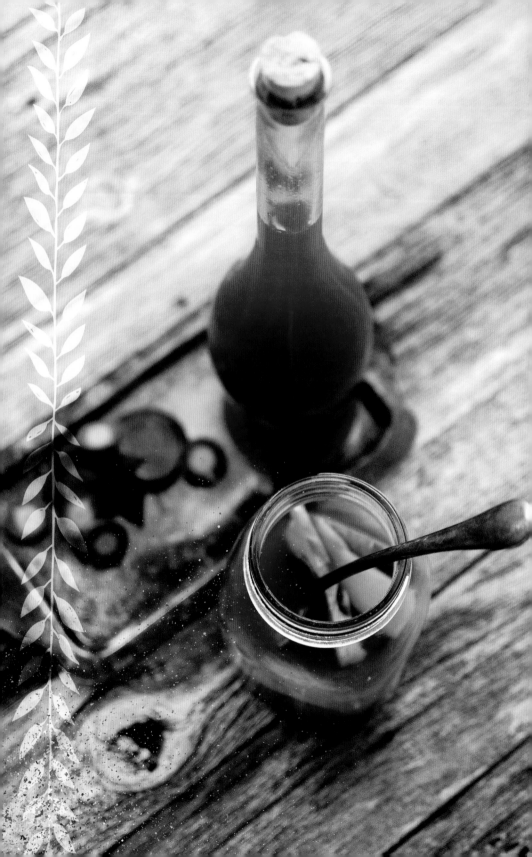

the labyrinth

*what the heart whispers*

chapter 26

*Walking with purpose means more than placing one foot in front of the other. It means moving with intention through your life. There are times when the clear expanse in front of you feels safe and familiar, and other times when the path is covered with leaves and hidden from you even when you kick the leaves aside. The spiral of your life twists and turns in mystery. Remember that you are not alone on this winding road; your own heart is your companion. Listen to the wisdom of this friend who has been with you since before the moment of your first breath.*

## FAMILY WELLNESS: *Intestinal Health*

The intestines are a labyrinth inside your physical body. Their ropy expanse holds the key to your underlying health. If your gut works properly, then all other systems can function at their best. On a basic level, your intestines capture vital nutrients from food. They support your immunity, hormones, and nervous system. The way your body breaks down food impacts your mental, physical, and emotional health.

Poor intestinal function has been linked to depression, fatigue, IBS, autoimmune disease, and inflammation.[69, 70] Various environmental factors can stress our gut health, including medications such as antibiotics and NSAIDS, although these may sometimes be necessary. Other stressors include processed foods, alcohol, caffeine, gluten, dairy products, and sugar. By minimizing these stressors and taking care of your gut, you are taking care of your whole body.

*Intestinal TLC to gently bring your intestines into balance*

- **Focus on eating whole, unprocessed foods.** Avoid, or at least reduce, foods that can cause intestinal stress such gluten, dairy products, sugar, and refined carbs.

- **Give your body time and rest to repair.** If your gut is damaged it can take 2–3 years to fully recover. So be kind to yourself, and generously give yourself enough time to heal.

- **Take extra nourishment** in the form of aloe vera, probiotics, and gut-friendly herbs including cinnamon and turmeric. Other great things to add to the diet are omega 3s, zinc, and vitamins A, C, and E.
- **Walking** is a nice, gentle movement that is great for giving the intestines a natural massage from the inside.

## SPIRITUAL APPLICATION: *Heart, Gut, and Mind*

Have you heard the phrase "trust your gut"? Or how about listening to a "gut feeling," or getting "butterflies in your stomach"? Many global medicinal traditions recognize a link between the heart, head, and gut. Some even say this relationship is the seat of our intuition. The vagus nerve, which connects the brain and the gut, relays a huge amount of information between the two—and in both directions. The gut has been called your "second brain" because of the intense and continuous amount of communication it regularly shares with your brain. Don't discount those messages from deep inside your body. In many cultures, your abdominal region is your real center, containing your roots and your core knowing. It is a place of purpose, strength, and presence.

## SOUL CHALLENGE: *Belly Breath*

Place your hands on your stomach, right below your belly button. Imagine your stomach is a balloon. When you inhale, expand your lungs and breathe all the way into your stomach. Your hands should lift a little as you fill with air. Once you are full, release your breath completely, allowing your hands to sink with the exhalation. After three rounds of this breathing, say the affirmation, "I trust my gut. My body is wise." Say it three times. Close the practice with a smile.

## GLOBAL APOTHECARY: *Kombucha—Ancient Probiotics*

Kombucha is a fermented drink, usually made from green or black tea. It has been around for over 2,000 years, although no one is quite sure where it originated. There is a long anecdotal history of kombucha curing many a serious illness. At the very least, it is wonderful for supporting great gut health, because the natural enzymes and probiotics deeply nourish the intestines. Besides helping digestion, kombucha has been found to assist liver detoxification and provide a good range of nutrients. It can be made at home by using a SCOBY (symbiotic colony of bacteria and yeast); or you can purchase it ready-made at your natural food store.[71, 72]

## Conjuring and Crafting

Supporting your gut health is easy by adding fun and interesting foods such as fermented fruits and vegetables. The fermentation process creates enzymes and natural probiotics that keep gut flora healthy.

---

### CHILDREN'S HERBAL BITTERS

*Offered by Sarah Josey at Golden Poppy Herbal Apothecary.*

As an herbalist, I often find that young children's complaints usually stem from one of two places—either their stomach hurts, or they are overly tired and their entire system is at its breaking point. This herbal bitters formula is great for helping both of these issues, as the herbs help soothe both the digestive and nervous systems.

Herbal bitters work by increasing the flow of digestive juices, to help break down food better, relieve gas and bloating, and gently improve elimination. The bitter flavor has been shown to stimulate the digestive tract from end to end, and using bitters before and after meals and anytime they are needed will greatly improve digestive health—and thus overall health.

The following recipe is easy to make, and will produce quite a bit of tincture. It is made with alcohol; however, the amount of alcohol contained in a single dose is about the same as in a very ripe banana. That said, you can make this with glycerin instead of alcohol, which will produce a very sweet remedy that kids will most likely enjoy; but it won't be as strong, medicinally. You can also mix up these herbs and keep them as a tea blend, to make and serve when needed.

**Note:** All amounts are by weight except the alcohol, measured by volume.

- Large glass Mason jar with lid
- Cheesecloth
- Blank label and pen
- Additional bottle for storage of tincture (about 8-ounce size)—you can use a Boston round bottle, or simply put it back in the Mason jar
- $3/5$ ounce chamomile flowers, dried
- $1/10$ ounce dried orange peels
- $1/10$ ounce dried lemon balm leaves
- $1/10$ ounce fennel seed
- 10 ounces organic vodka, brandy, or glycerin

Place all herbs into a large glass jar, and shake well to mix. Cover with the alcohol or glycerin. Seal and shake well again. Label with the name, ingredients, and date. Place jar in a dark place. Shake daily for 6 weeks. At the end of 6 weeks, strain the herbs out of the alcohol through cheesecloth, squeezing out as much liquid as possible. Compost the herbs. Save the newly created tincture in a bottle of choice, being sure to label it with the name and ingredients.

Mix ½ teaspoon of the tincture into a small amount of water, and drink before and after meals, or when there is a tummy ache.

**Please note:** A persistent tummy ache in a child may be a sign of deeper trouble, so please be sure to check with your pediatrician if you are concerned.

---

## HARVEST KVASS

Kvass is a traditional fermented beet juice. It can be an acquired taste, so to make the natural benefits more palatable we've added sweet carrots and spicy ginger.

- 2-quart jar
- 4-pint plastic bottles for storing the kvass
- Plastic strainer
- Coffee filter, or small piece of cotton cloth
- Rubber band
- 2 beets, thinly sliced
- 4 carrots, thinly sliced
- 1 thumb-sized piece of ginger
- 2 teaspoons salt
- ¼ cup whey (the liquid off the top of a good organic, whole-fat yogurt; to make dairy-free kvass, simply use 4 teaspoons of salt instead of two, and omit the whey)
- About 2 quarts pure water
- 4 teaspoons raw local honey (optional)

Layer the beets, carrots, and ginger in a sterile 2-quart jar. Sprinkle salt and whey over the veggies. Fill the jar with water, leaving about an inch of space at the top. Cover and give it a vigorous shake to mingle all the ingredients and dissolve the salt. Remove lid, and cover with coffee filter or cloth, keeping it in place with a rubber band.

Keep in a warm spot for about 2–4 days, and start to taste it after 48 hours to see whether it has fermented to your liking. The longer you leave the vegetables soaking, the more sour

they will become. Once it
tastes right for you, strain
the liquid from the veg-
gies. You can compost
the veggies at this point,
or you can reserve about
1 cup of the liquid as a
starter and use it to make
a second batch with the

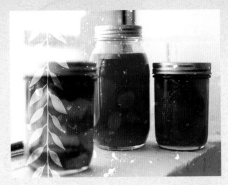

same veggies, simply combining the veggies with the cup of
reserved starter and topping with water.

   If you like your tart vegetable juice fizzy, you can do a second
fermentation. Place your kvass liquid in bottles with 1 teaspoon of honey per bottle, and let it ferment for another
24–48 hours. Plastic bottles are best for this, with a short fermentation time, because if you leave glass bottles too long they
can explode from the expanding gas created by the breakdown
of sugar.

## FIZZY FERMENTED AUTUMN FRUITS

This recipe can be made seasonally with whatever fruit is available. It is briefly fermented to add a blissful fizz. It is great as a
topping on yogurt, pancakes, and ice cream.

- Pint-size jar
- Wooden spoon or stirring stick
- 2 plums
- 1 apple
- 10 blackberries
- 3 Tablespoons fresh whey (the liquid off the top of a good,
  organic, whole-fat yogurt)
- 2 Tablespoons raw local honey
- Pure water

Place berries in jar. Chop other fruit and place in jar. Mix whey and honey, and pour over fruit. Top with water, and use wooden stick to stir and release air. Make sure fruit is completely covered in liquid. Cover jar, and leave at room temperature for 48 hours. Then drain liquid.

Serve over yogurt or pancakes or ice cream. Yum!

## Pairings

- Belly Massage: Ampuku, Mizan, and Mayan are all types of massage that focus on abdomens.

- Walking a Labyrinth: A meditative practice of walking with purpose and intention.

- Intestinal Health Ally: Probiotics are a great boost, especially if you recently have been ill and/or taken antibiotics. Studies are now linking specific strains of probiotics to specific medical conditions.

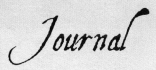

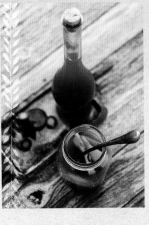

As we spiral into the dark nights of the year, pause to consider where this path of healing and well-being is taking you. Do you know what the next step is?

_____

_____

_____

_____

_____

_____

_____

_____

_____

_____

_____

_____

_____

_____

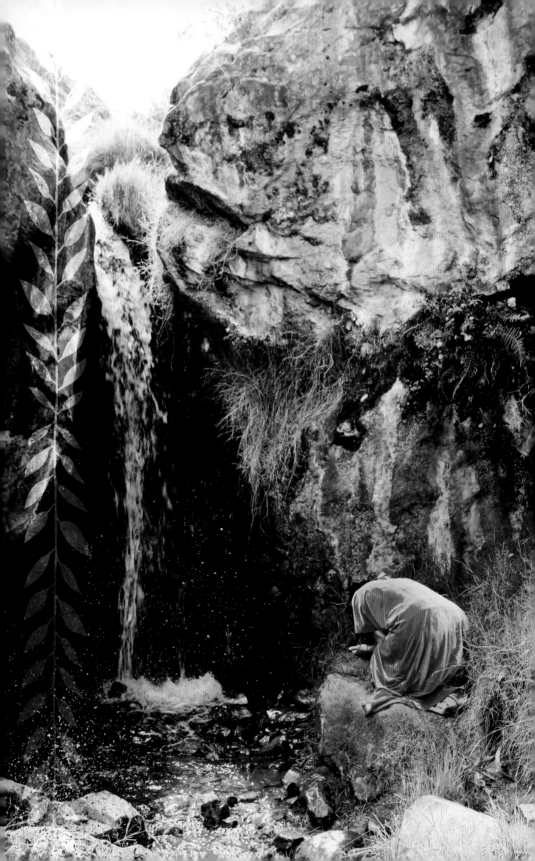

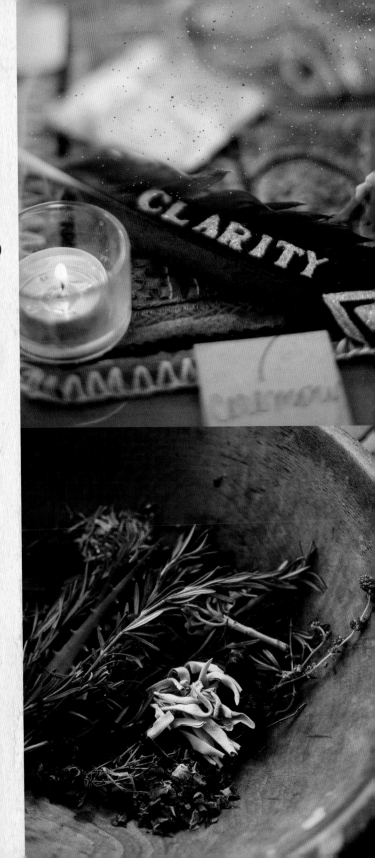

*enchanting intentions*

# spell

chapter 27

*Linger a moment in the last shadows of autumn's fading sunset. This golden light summons you to step over the threshold of fall into winter, and into the home of mystery and Spirit. To "spell" is to link letters together to form intentional words that will soar into the universal void, and eventually land on your destiny.*

*Words resonate from your heart; they are projected through your lips to communicate your thoughts and your dreams. Words shape your needs, desires, and intentions into forms that take on their own life. In the oldest practices, forming words with pure intention was part of bridging the vision of a dream to the reality of action. In this way, spells are an act of creation.*

## FAMILY WELLNESS: *Story and Word Medicine*

One of the most ancient forms of medicine, handed down from generation to generation, is the art of storytelling. The elders have used it to help heal people, communities, and global vision. Folklore has been held and passed down with sacred care by the writers, poets, artists, medicine folks, and shamans of civilizations, and it is how we know much of what we do today.

Ancient remedies shared in wooded groves, childbirth traditions, whispered secrets of the divine feminine, moon magic, and blood mysteries, plant and animal medicines, and energy healings—all of these came to us from stories shared by keepers of the wisdom who honored and guarded them with deep care. Much of what is in this book came from ancient lands and handed-down lore from wise ancestors unknown, from days past when ritual and ceremony were the healing modalities of choice, and the plant world and Mother Earth held all of the wisdom we needed.

This community medicine begins in your own heart and mind. Your body and soul hear everything you say. They vibrate with each word you speak, and resonate with your thoughts. The language you use to describe your state of being and your experience of health and the world is a key part of achieving wellness.

Often, however, with health challenges, the words you speak are exactly the opposite of what you want to achieve. For example, in the medical world of fertility treatment, terms such as "hostile uterus" or "lazy sperm," or even "trying to conceive" are repeated endlessly. In pregnancy, the ever-popular "contractions are so painful" is a recurring chant. You may use phrases like "I have a weak immune system" or "I am always getting sick," or maybe even "I am so depressed!"

These may be accurate descriptions of your experience—but they are also potent negative mantras. Are these the kinds of words that you want going into your every cell, over and over? Instead of making negative judgments about your body's wisdom, try reframing your words into something truthful and accepting. You could say, "I have a powerful body" instead of "a hostile uterus," or simply, "I trust my body's wisdom." Another example might be "My body is working hard right now" instead of "I have a weak immune system." These alternatives are clear acknowledgments without negative connotations.

Words are medicine. Words linked together become spells and stories. Taking this even further, stories are how people attach meaning to events. Once we understand that we are in control of that meaning, we become powerful creators of our own realities.

What gift of positive word medicine will you give yourself today? How are you using your words to shape your world?

## SPIRITUAL APPLICATION: *Positive Habits*

You have the power to create positive habits in your life by activating your intentions, words, and actions. Creating effective positive habits means taking the practices of word medicine and affirmations into actual reality. The first step is to get clear about your goal—maybe you want to be more generous, or to eat healthier. The next step is to see yourself clearly living that goal. Once you see the steps you need to get there, it is time to implement them.

## SOUL CHALLENGE: *Positive Creation*

Choose a new positive habit to start in your life. Use a daily affirmation as a reminder to trigger the new behavior. Then do it every day for an entire month; this establishes a consistent pattern that will create soul and body memory. Finally, at the end of the month, solidify the habit by acknowledging and honoring your accomplishment.

## GLOBAL APOTHECARY: *Connecting with the Elements*

Elemental powers play a significant role in many global healing traditions. In Traditional Chinese Medicine, there are five elements that flow with the seasons of the passing year. The Water element is expressed in winter, Wood in spring, Fire in early summer, Earth in the harvest time of late summer, and Metal in autumn. Native American medicine also uses the elements of Earth, Air, Fire, and Water, as do traditional Celtic practices. In pagan traditions, Earth sits in the north and represents grounding and stability; Air sits in the east and represents Divine Mind and our thoughts; Fire sits in the south and represents our will and passions; and Water sits in the west and represents the flow of our emotions. Ayurveda, aboriginal medicine, and South American medicine also acknowledge the elements in some way.

When you connect with the elements, you are deepening your relationship with nature. Exploring the fluidity of Water, the heat of Fire, the strength of the Earth, the movement of Air, the precision of Metal—and how the memory in crystals weaves these archetypes into the fabric of your daily life—brings you more into the natural balance of holistic living.

## Conjuring and Crafting

Here are some spells and potions to diversify your medicine cupboard stores. Infuse each ingredient with the soft whispers of your soul. Layer actions, intentions, and words together in the time-honored practice of spellcraft, to bestir the most potent magic of your creations.

# BLACK SALT

Black Salt has been used for centuries as a protection against all forms of negative energy. It can also be used for banishing toxic folks you truly do not want in your space. Salt is a crystal, and therefore is able to form and hold energy. An old wives' tale is that salt bends to our will, and will do anything we ask of it.

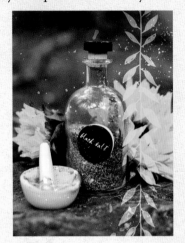

Black salt is extremely easy to make, and it takes only a couple of minutes to throw together a batch to last you for a while. This is ceremonial salt, so while you are making it, hold the intention of protection for your home, your family, and yourself.

- 1 cup sea salt or kosher salt
- ½ cup finely ground charcoal
- ½ cup finely ground black pepper
- 10 drops rosemary essential oil

Use a mortar and pestle to grind all of the ingredients together. Store in a jar. Hold the jar in your hands and say a **Black Salt Protection Spell:**

*Black Salt of ancient and wise course,*
*Keep away all negativity and stray energies without remorse.*
*Black Salt, blessed with magic from Mother Earth,*
*Keep me safe, energetically clear, and full of mirth.*
*I charge you with intention of high vibration, love, and heart,*
*And ask, for the highest good of all concerned, that you are now activated and ready to start!*

Sprinkle Black Salt along the threshold of your doorway to keep your home safe. The idea is that it will keep bad energies and people from wanting to enter your home. You can even sprinkle it along the edge of your yard, if you want your entire property to be protected. If you need protection from bad dreams, or wish to rid your bed of negative energies, sprinkle a little black salt under your bed, or keep it in a bowl near or under your bed.

Once your black salt has served its purpose, be sure to throw it out. It has already used up its charge, and therefore holds no more protective energies. If you try to reuse it, there is no guarantee that it will work.

---

## MARIGOLD TEA

Marigolds are the flower of the season, and are filled with marvelous healing properties as well as brilliant beauty! The marigold flower is amazing for overall health. The tea purifies the blood, and the plant also has antiseptic, anti-inflammatory, and antibacterial properties, and is excellent in healing burns, corns, and calluses.

- 2 teaspoons dried marigolds
- 1 whole star anise
- 1 whole clove

Dry out the buds in a well-ventilated area (don't dry them in the oven, even on low heat). Hang them upside-down and keep them out of direct sunlight—after a couple of weeks, they will have dried thoroughly. (If you do not want to dry them yourself, most health food and herbal remedies stores carry dried marigolds.)

Boil 1 liter of water. Put 2 teaspoons of marigolds in the boiling water, add spices, turn off the heat, and cover. Allow the petals to infuse for 10 minutes. Cool, then drink 2–3 cups a day.

*Pairings*

- Book: *Encyclopedia of 5,000 Spells* by Judika Illes—a practical and timeless resource for those called to spellwork.

- Class: Sacred Elements with Jessica Booth: an intimate exploration of your connection to the Elements.

- Crystal: Pyrite—fantastic for supporting positive thinking and positive word medicine.

# *Journal*

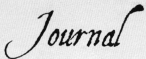

Take some time to play with spells,
and journal what comes up in your
conjuring.

_____

_____

_____

_____

_____

_____

_____

_____

_____

_____

_____

_____

_____

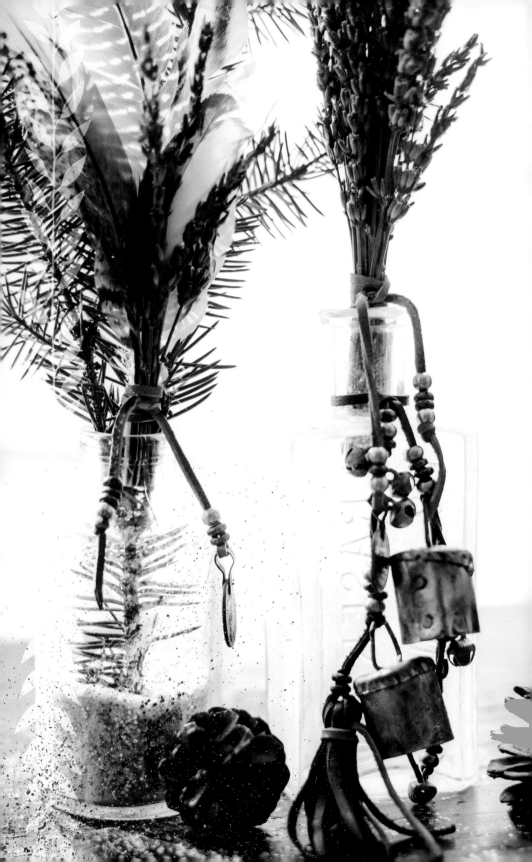

# PART FOUR

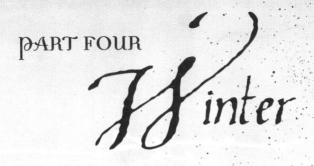

## Winter

Winter is the province of mystery

Where you coil into your deepest cave

And find your treasure lying dormant within.

The stars keep watch, enraptured by the auroral scintillations

Of those dreamers who dare to wander the lands and skies

Of their imaginations unrestrained and unfiltered.

Shift into the dark season,

And follow the timeless path of Inanna.

Descend into the underworld,

Where all things gestate before rebirth.

Be formed and reformed in the Great Mother's cauldron.

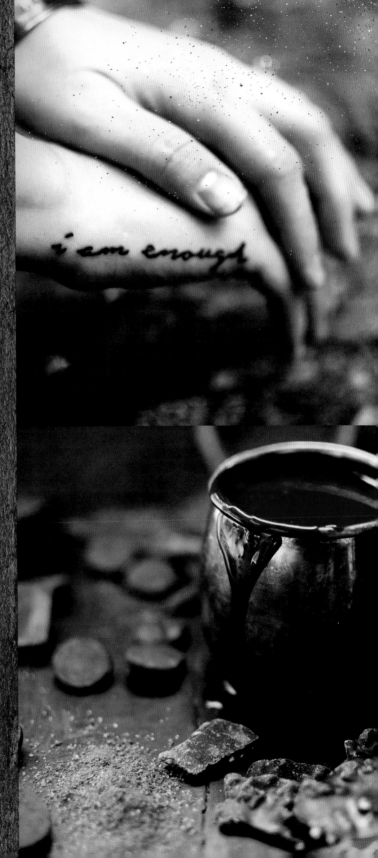

midnight *reflecting the inner landscape*

chapter 28

In the hushed hours of winter, you can befriend deep introspection and the stillness of quiet hours by the hearth. In the silent residence of this sacred mystery,
you embrace the closing season of the year, where all pretense is dropped and the
opportunity to excavate your forgotten bones and hidden desires stirs. You dance at
the borderlands of memory and release.

In these surrendering hours, travel the road to the underworld. Allow yourself
to fall into winter's slow dance, and move to the grace of this slower pace. Only the
trees that lose all their leaves and stand bare in the long, dark winter can emerge
fully revitalized in the spring.

## FAMILY WELLNESS: *Depression*

The grey weight of depression touches so many people today. Nearly
sixteen million people in the U.S. alone experience depression each
year. Young people under the age of twenty-four have a one-in-four
chance of suffering at least one episode of depression.

There are certain known triggers for depression; these include
genetics, brain chemistry, hormones, and stress situations such as
trauma, grief, or financial issues—but none of these are needed to
call the beast to the table. Depression can be triggered by any loss of
identity, such as through poverty, exposure to violence, or simply by
expectations not meeting day-to-day reality.

Ironically, depression takes an incredible amount of energy, and
the person experiencing it often feels drained, exhausted, and disas-
sociated from day-to-day life.

*So how do you support someone with depression?*

- **Acknowledge what is going on.** You don't have to know exactly
  how someone is feeling to understand that they are in pain. Nam-
  ing hard feelings like sadness, grief, anger, and depression are an
  important step in moving through them. Until the hard stuff is
  brought into the light, it hangs around festering in the shadows.

- **Be present.** You cannot "fix" someone else's depression; you are not responsible for other people's happiness or outlook on life. A great tool for supporting anyone is simply practicing empathic listening skills. This kind of listening comes from the heart, and is meant for understanding rather than responding.

- **Take care of yourself.** This means to set clear boundaries about what you can and cannot give, to not take things personally, and to be sure you yourself have a support network. Looking after yourself will give you the energy you need to support your loved one without draining your own personal resources.

- **Go for a walk in nature.** Exercise and nature have been proven to reduce stress and depression. Spending time outside and getting the body moving are simple, constructive steps. Nature is not only the plant kingdom; research has shown that spending time with animals can also calm anxiety and soothe feelings of isolation.

- **Help them find support that works for them.** There are many different support systems out there for depression—therapists, counseling, support groups, acupuncture, bodywork, and somatic experiencing, to name a few. Ask your loved one if they would like you to help research viable options.

- **Eat well.** Since nutrition plays a role in brain chemistry and hormonal health, eating a balanced diet high in omega 3s and superfoods can help stabilize the mood. Preparing nourishing foods for your loved one can be a huge support.

- **Stay positive.** It is okay to remind your loved one that they won't feel like this forever. You can acknowledge and validate their experience without making it your own. Being around your high vibration will help them see that the whole world is not grey.

- **Certain plants can be a valuable support** if you or a loved one is dealing with depression. Make sure to check with your care provider before taking any herbs.[73, 74]

Studies of St. John's Wort show that it may be beneficial for mild depression.[75] *Xiao Yao San (Xiao Yao Wan),* also called "Free and Easy

Wanderer," is a traditional Chinese herbal combination, classically made with six ingredients: *Bupleurum* root, white peony root, *Angelica sinensis* root *(dong quai)*, *Poria*, white *Atractylodes*, and licorice root. Variations on this formula may include mint, ginger, or other herbs. This ancient formula has shown promising results in studies in supporting depression.[76, 77]

## SPIRITUAL APPLICATION: *Empathy*

Empathy is defined as being able to feel what another is feeling. This is the ability not only to put yourself in someone else's shoes, but to feel the experience from their perspective. It is a connected understanding of another's experience.

## SOUL CHALLENGE: *Empathic Listening*

Empathic listening seeks to understand before being understood. Being a good listener means you are neutral, open, and attentive. You do not need to give advice, or fix the issue. Remember that empathy means to feel "as" someone, not "with" someone. Listening skills are a life's work, so be patient with yourself and play with these tools.

- **Listen first, speak little.** There is no need to interrupt or talk over someone.
- **Allow their story to unfold** in its own way.
- **Be attentive to their language.** Stay out of your own head, and avoid planning out your response in advance.
- **Allow, witness, and see the person and all of their feelings.** You are not there to fix, teach, or problem-solve.
- **Mirror back to the person, with their own language, what they are saying.** If you do not know what something means, ask for further clarification.

# GLOBAL APOTHECARY:
## *Energetic Balancing Visualization*

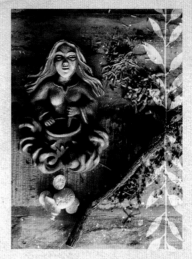

Energy balancing is a practice to bring harmony to your subtle spiritual systems. Here is one simple method, based on the classic "cosmic-orbit" meditation.

Imagine in your mind's eye a beautiful, glowing ball of light beaming softly at the base of your spine. This ball of light, shining right at the lowest point of your back, feels warm, safe, and happy. It can glow any color you like—white, gold, violet, blue, green, yellow, orange, red, indigo, or like a shining rainbow crystal with a little of every color softly pulsing out from its center.

The lustrous ball of light begins to move up your spine, very gently and very slowly, right up the center of your back. As it moves, the ball of light shines gently, warmly, and safely into your body and out around you. The ball infuses every cell in your body, and every molecule around you, with its warm, loving light. Everywhere the light touches feels calm, relaxed, and healthy.

The ball now reaches the place on your back that is exactly opposite your belly button. It pauses here a moment, sending out an extra beam of love and health to your body. This little glowing ball loves every cell in you. It loves you in your entirety, wholly and completely.

The vibrant ball of warmth and love drifts slowly up your spine, moving up past each of your ribs, relaxing and soothing each muscle, bone, and cell as it passes. Up and up it gently floats, now pausing a moment at the back of your neck.

Drifting up further, the shining ball passes over the back of your head, coming to a stop right at the top of your head, where it becomes infused with a brilliant white-gold light, like the light of the stars. The golden-white light feels amazing—it imbues you with feelings of serenity. The beautiful light soaks into every cell in your whole body, and into the very air and space around you. Just enjoy these feelings of peace.

When you are ready, tell the little ball to begin moving again. It floats gently now to your forehead, and then falls softly to the tip of your nose. It moves down to your lips, where you open your mouth and swallow it. The orb tastes sparkly, and a little fizzy. The light is now beaming out from inside of you. It glides down your throat and stops at your heart, where it begins to pulse, slowly and softly, in time with your heart's easy, natural rhythm. As you feel the illumination soak into your core, your breathing becomes even more relaxed, and you are instilled with a deep, restful feeling.

Gently, the ball slips down further into your belly, just below your belly button, imparting every part of you, every part of each cell, with a soft, loving, golden-white light. You feel so tranquil, so calm, and so safe, from deep in your center. The light touches everywhere, from fingertips to toes, inside and outside, and even into the spaces all around you. You are one with your inner light.

## Conjuring and Crafting

### HOMEMADE "TO-THE-RESCUE" FLOWER ESSENCE

Bach Flower Remedies' traditional Rescue Remedy is a combination of five flowers to soothe trauma, shock, grief, fear, and pain. Over the course of this year, you have acquired and made several flower essences, and this one will be your own bespoke emergency essence.

Choose 5 flower essences that most resonate with you, and add 5 drops of each to a bottle filled with 2/3 organic vodka and ⅓ pure spring water. Make a beautiful label called "To the Rescue." Use during any emotional turbulence.

## RAY-OF-LIGHT MISTER

Use your new To-the-Rescue Flower Essence (above) in this gentle, calming, and uplifting mister.

- 3-ounce mister bottle
- 3 drops flower essence (choose 1 from these): To-the-Rescue (above), gorse, or honeysuckle
- 10 drops bergamot essential oil
- 10 drops rose geranium essential oil
- 5 drops clary sage essential oil
- 2½ ounces pure spring water
- 1 teaspoon solvent (vodka, witch hazel, or vanilla extract)
- Small tumble-stone smoky quartz crystal

Mix oils, flower essences, and solvent together. Add water and crystal. Leave on your altar to charge it. When you feel it is ready, put liquid in misting bottle and mist around space and your aura as needed.

## SACRED CACAO DRINK AND CEREMONY

Chocolate is made from the cacao plant. Its scientific name, *Theobroma cacao,* means "food of the gods." Cacao is a superfood, containing more than 300 nutrients. It has many properties; it is stimulating, antibacterial, antioxidant, and supportive of the neurotransmitters and circulatory system.[78, 79]

Raw cacao stimulates the release of love hormones and a feeling of euphoria. It elevates the vibrations of body and soul. Many people who work with the spirit of this plant have found that it very much wants to help us shift to a higher state of consciousness. South American ancestors who keep this wisdom take cacao in a more traditional form that has been known to have euphoric and spiritual effects. This may be due to the potent neurotransmitters in the pure form of this plant. If you enjoy this ceremony, please seek out an ethical source of ceremonial-grade cacao from South America and the cacao wisdom-keepers.

*For the cacao drink:*

- 2 ounces best-quality raw dark chocolate OR 2 ounces raw cacao powder
- ⅛–¼ teaspoon chili powder
- 1 teaspoon cinnamon
- Honey, to taste (optional)
- 1 cup water

As you stir each ingredient into this recipe, ask for guidance and blessings from the Cacao Deva.

*If using the dark chocolate:* Begin to melt the chocolate over low heat, stirring constantly. Once the chocolate has begun to melt, add in all the ingredients except the water. Warm the water. Once the chocolate is melted and the spices well combined, whisk the warm water into the chocolate paste. You may need to add a little more water to get a thick, drinkable consistency.

*If using the raw cacao powder:* Heat the water to simmering. Add in all the other ingredients, and whisk well.

*For the ceremony:*

Light a candle, and hold your cup. With respect, ask the Spirit of the Cacao to bless this medicine you have made. Sip your brew, and trace its warmth through your body and soul. Be open to what comes up for you. Notice any emotions, thoughts, or memories. Close the ceremony by thanking the cacao, and putting out the candle.

## Pairings

- Plant Ally: Gorse flower essence—brings a ray of light and hope to a heavy heart.

- Crystal Ally: Carnelian—grounding, warming, joyful, and balancing to the sacral chakra.

- Resource: Suicide Prevention Lifeline 1-800-273-TALK (-8255). It is okay to reach out and get support. Sometimes help is just a phone call away.

# *Journal*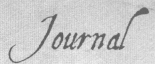

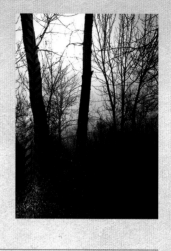

Play with empathic listening this week.
Use this space to explore what that means
to you, and how you can incorporate it
into your life.

_____

_____

_____

_____

_____

_____

_____

_____

_____

_____

_____

_____

_____

_____

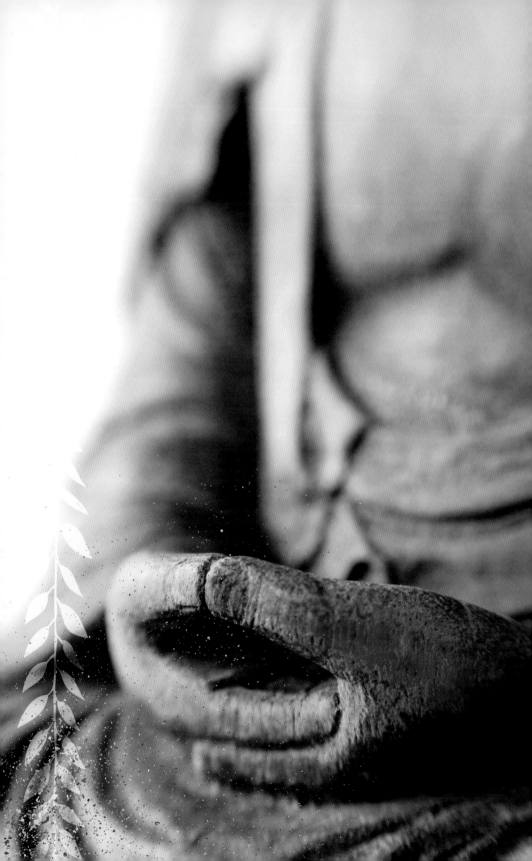

# contemplation

*peace & bliss*

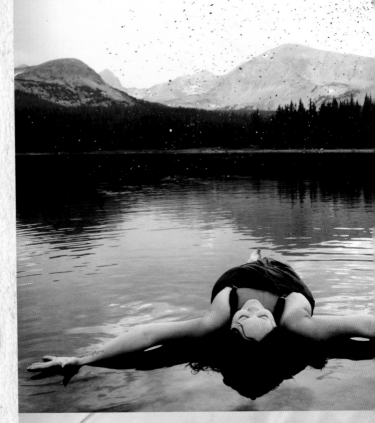

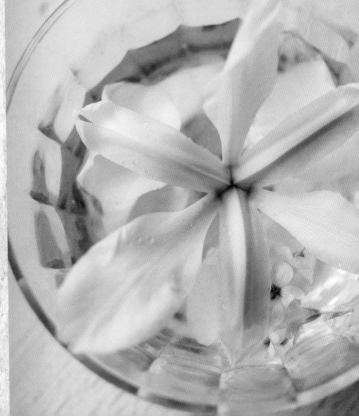

## chapter 29

*Winter is a slow spooling-inward of nature's energy, and your own energy fol-*
*lows this cue. Outside of the holidays, it is a still and restful time when people*
*yearn to cozy up indoors. The long nights invite internal processes. Contempla-*
*tion is self-awareness, a reflective and integrative exploration of your heart and*
*life's purpose. Approach your inner sanctuary with neutrality, and enter the gates*
*of your soul temple with reverence. Be in awe at the wonder of you.*

## FAMILY WELLNESS: *Anxiety*

Worry is a normal response to stressful situations. However, anxiety that is recurring or persists for a long time can be debilitating.
More and more people in today's busy world experience anxiety at
some point. If this a consistent problem for you, do not face it alone.
Reach out to your care provider and your family, and get some support. In many ways, tools that work for depression can help with anxiety, although the two conditions are different. Here are some coping
skills to practice when the panic hits:[80]

· **Slow Down.** You are allowed to take a break from things that raise
  your stress levels. Examples of slowing down are walks in nature,
  yoga, meditation, or massage. Do things that you enjoy.

· **Eat well.** Eat nourishing foods throughout the day, as this can help
  balance your energy and mood.

· **Focus on your breathing.** Take deep breaths, and really be present
  in your body.

· **Practice good sleep habits.** This one speaks for itself.

· **Practice acceptance.** Work on accepting that you cannot control every outcome, and that everything does not need to be perfect.

· **Work with plants:** Some popular natural remedies such as passion
  flower, lemon balm, and white chestnut can help ease anxiety. Please
  check with your care provider if you decide to try these herbs.

  · **Passionflower**—studies show this plant is very helpful in reducing
    anxiety and insomnia. Be aware that it may cause drowsiness.[81]

- **Lemon balm**—especially good for anxiety when combined with hops and chamomile.[82]
- **White chestnut flower essence**—helps to reduce intrusive or repetitive thoughts, and is very calming to the mind.

## SPIRITUAL APPLICATION: *Happiness*

*The present moment is the only moment available to us, and it is the door to all moments.*
—THICH NHAT HANH

Happiness is a sweet contentment that comes from inside your soul. The key to this well-being lies in your own personal satisfaction with who you are and how you interact with the world. Happiness is not a commodity to be sought after; it lives within you, and can only be tapped with an elevated consciousness. Align your life goals with your true soul path, and happiness flourishes.

## SOUL CHALLENGE: *Find Your Bliss*

Find your bliss by meditating on the times this week when you lived as you have been called. This means noticing the moments where your actions, soul, and heart were all in alignment. Begin by making a list of actions you took in any given situation that made you feel good. These might include creating art, an act of generosity, or keeping your high vibration when things were hard. You may find a pattern, or a common link between your actions and your happiness.

## GLOBAL APOTHECARY: *Shiatsu*

Shiatsu is a Japanese massage therapy based on a combination of Traditional Chinese Medicine and Western physiology and pathology. The word *shiatsu* means "finger pressure." It is a full-body massage practice that supports balance and wellness in the body's energy systems—and it feels great. Shiatsu is a great complementary therapy that combines well with Western medicine.

## CALM ESSENCE

Create an essence to soothe tension and anxiety. Choose a tree, plant, or crystal that calls to your heart. Ask Mother Nature for what you need most, and she will answer.

- Glass bowl
- Piece of cheesecloth or strainer
- Pint-size Mason jar (to store mother essence)
- 1 cup pure spring water or sacred water (from a holy, pure source)
- Nature item to support your grounding work; plant materials are best gathered alive and at the peak of their growth
- 1 cup organic vodka or brandy

Follow the "Making a Flower Essence" instructions in Chapter 1. Take 1 drop on the tongue, or 3 drops diluted in a glass of water and sipped throughout the day.

## PEACE TEA

A sweet and soothing blend for anxious spirits and tired souls.

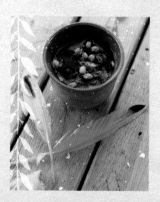

- ½ cup dried lemon balm
- ¼ cup dried passion flower
- ¼ cup dried lavender blossoms
- ¼ cup dried jasmine flowers
- ¼ cup dried rose petals
- ¼ cup dried catnip

Simply mix the herbs together, and store them in a sealed jar. When needed, brew using 1 heaping Tablespoon in a teapot for about 10 minutes. Strain and serve. Sweeten with honey if you like.

---

## BLISS STICK

A favorite combination to infuse bliss into your daily life.

- ⅓-ounce (10-ml.) rollerball tube with ball and lid
- Plastic pipette
- Small bowl or measuring jug
- Just under ⅓ ounce (9 ml.) of carrier oil such as rose oil or almond oil
- 10 drops benzoin oil
- 10 drops rose geranium essential oil
- 10 drops grapefruit essential oil
- 10 drops sandalwood essential oil
- 3 drops strawberry flower essence

Mix together carrier oil, essential oils, and flower essence in the bowl or measuring jug. Use the plastic pipette to transfer the oil mixture into the rollerball.

Roll on back of neck, pulse points, and temples (around the hairline only—avoid contact with eyes). You can also rub it into your hands, cup hands near your nose, and inhale.

### Pairings

- Book: *Wherever You Go, There You Are: Mindfulness Meditation in Everyday Life* by Jon Kabat-Zinn. A popular bestselling introduction to mindfulness practices, which can be a great support to people with anxiety.
- Activity: *T'ai chi*—a moving-meditation practice from Asia that balances energy, provides exercise, and is conducive to a relaxed brain state.

# Journal

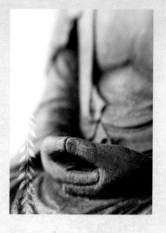

Make yourself a warming cup of Peace Tea (above), and contemplate the bliss of your soul. Use this space to free-associate about what makes you happy.

_____

_____

_____

_____

_____

_____

_____

_____

_____

_____

_____

_____

_____

_____

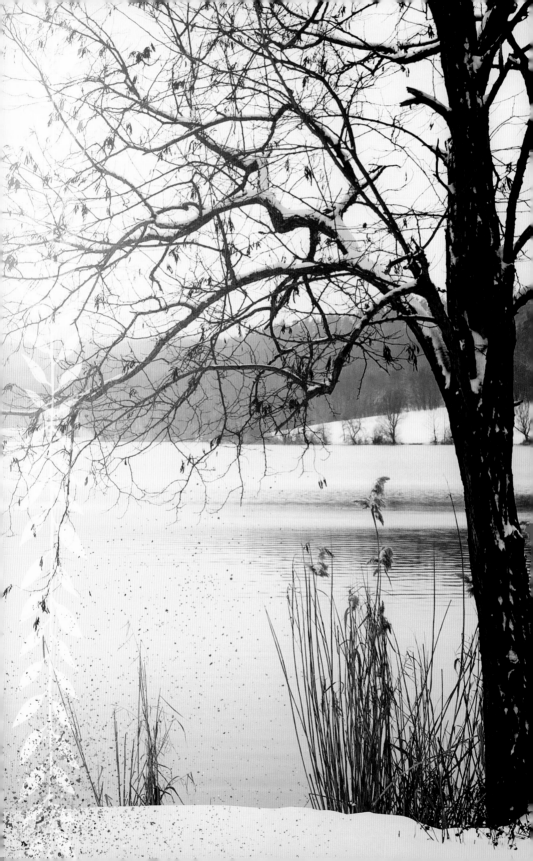

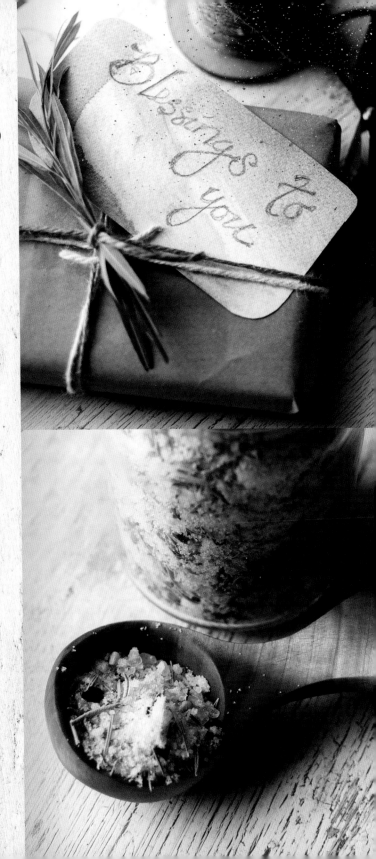

# winter solstice

## all the blessings

chapter 30

*Stretching deep into the vast and timeless sea of stars, the quiet night beckons with pristine calm. The immense expanse of dark rests heavy on the cold span of the winter landscape. The Earth is sleeping; the heavens keep watch. Suddenly, a streak of light splits the potent peace of the blackness. The sun has returned—it is the moment that the tide of the year changes and the light begins to be restored. Midnight turns into dawn, winter to spring, and the wheel spins again. Lift your heart and rejoice; it is the season of illumination.*

## FAMILY WELLNESS: *Lungs Inspiring Health*

Lungs physically govern your inspiration and exhalation. They oxygenate your blood, and play a role in your immune system. Winter can be a challenging time for lung health, with seasonal sniffles, coughs, and wheezes making them work overtime. The American Lung Association suggests the following tips for keeping your lungs working at their best.

- **Avoid lung stressors** such as smoking, exposure to secondhand smoke, air pollution, and radon in the home.

- **Follow good hygiene practices** to prevent infection. These include washing your hands, good oral hygiene, covering your mouth when you sneeze or cough, and staying home if you are ill.

- **Exercise** helps build strong lungs. This includes taking up a breathing practice such as meditation or yoga.

Some global traditions that support good lung health are salt pipes and oil-pulling. Salt pipes are clay or porcelain pipes filled with healing salts. To use them, you pull mineral-enriched air into your lungs through salt in the pipe. This salt therapy is based on the time-honored European practice of spending time in salt caves for respiratory issues. Salt pipes have anecdotally been known to improve lung wellness for those with asthma.

Oil-pulling, an Ayurvedic tradition, is the practice of swishing oil, usually sesame or sunflower, around your mouth, or holding it under your tongue, for about twenty minutes, to pull out bacteria and germs.

## SPIRITUAL APPLICATION: *Completing Cycles*

Winter Solstice, the longest night of the year, is a celebration of the rebirth of sun. Once this night is over, the daylight lingers a little longer with each passing day. It marks the coming end of the winter, although the effects of the light won't be felt for some time yet. Now is the time to honor the completion of your own cycles. Say goodbye to old projects, tasks, and feelings, and welcome in the light of the new year.

## SOUL CHALLENGE: *Completion*

Begin to prepare the fertile ground of your soul for new plantings by honoring and clearing away the old that remains from last year's cycle. This could be as simple as writing your accomplishments down and burning them, symbolizing their completion. Or it could be a focused assessment of tasks not yet completed, to decide whether they are worth taking forward into next spring's plantings.

## GLOBAL APOTHECARY: *Hand Chakras*

Hand chakras are a part of the minor chakra system. These swirling vortices of energy reside in the center of your palms. The hand chakras open to healing energy, allowing it to pass through your hands and flow out into the world. It is thought that the left palm is primarily for receiving, and the right palm for giving, although each have some capacity for both.

When your palm chakras are open and in balance, you can feel the energy just by raising your hands and bringing them close together. As they get closer, before the palms touch, see if you can sense any pulsating vibrations. This force can feel warm or cool, or like magnets pulsing against each other. This subtle resistance is the pooling of energy between your palms. "Barefoot breathing" (see Chapter 34) with your hands in prayer position, or placing your hands directly on the Earth, are wonderful ways to cleanse and balance your hand chakras.

# Conjuring and Crafting

Handcrafted goodies make heartfelt gifts for this season of giving.

---

## HERB-INFUSED SALTS

Double the recipes, and give these tasty salts as gifts to your friends and family.

### Rosemary and Lemon Salt

- Two 6-ounce jars
- 8 ounces sea salt
- 2 ounces rosemary
- 2 ounces lemon zest
- 1 ounce chili flakes
- 1 ounce garlic granules

Combine all ingredients in a bowl. Mix well. Pack into jars, and label them. Use in cooking to replace plain salt.

### Spiced Salts

- Two 6-ounce jars
- 8 ounces sea salt
- 2 ounces ground cumin
- 2 ounces ground coriander
- 1 ounce ground paprika
- 1 ounce ground allspice

Combine all ingredients in a bowl. Mix well. Pack into jars, and label them. Use in cooking to replace plain salt.

## HOLLY AND PINE BLESSING WATER

Holly and pine are sacred in Celtic traditions, and are of seasonal significance this time of year. With the right intention, though, any plant can be used to make blessing water.

- Quart jar
- Pure spring water
- Holly, harvested with the plant's permission
- Pine, harvested with the plant's permission
- 3 drops of your "To-the-Rescue" Flower Essence (from Chapter 28)

Fill the jar with holly, pine, and flower essence. Add water to cover everything. Leave for 3 days on an altar or in your sacred medicine space. Then strain the plants out, and compost their remains.

Use this Blessing Water in your protection and blessing spells. You may also bless your home and the people in it by sprinkling it around your house with prayers and positive intentions. Gift back to Mother Earth anything that is left over. There are no preservatives in this mixture, so it will not last long.

## YULE LOG CEREMONY

"Yule" is the Celtic name for the Winter Solstice celebration. The traditional Yule log is a piece of wood burned with sacred intent. Often it is decorated with a ribbon, berries, and handwritten wishes for the New Year. This is essentially a New Year's celebration, as the returning light means the cycle has transitioned.

- A lighter, or a fragment from last year's Yule log (if this is your first year, remember to keep a piece for next year)
- A piece of wood about a foot long, ideally from nature and taken with permission and reverence
- Ribbon, pine, holly berries, strips of paper, and natural decorating materials
- A safe place for a burning ember, and also for a bonfire
- Enough tinder and kindling to light the Yule log
- One candle for each person
- A seasonal story

Use the ribbon, pine, and holly berries to decorate the Yule log. Write your New Year wishes on the paper, and tuck them into the ribbon on the log. After you have decorated the Yule log during the afternoon, set up your safe space for a bonfire.

After dinner, extinguish all of the lights in the house except for one burning ember. Give one candle to each person, and sit in a circle. We like to use long candles fitted into paper cups to catch hot-wax drips. The candles are unlit except for those around the storyteller.

The storyteller shares a seasonal story. Some years, it is the traditional story of the rebirth of the sun; or you could tell the nativity tale if you like, or choose another traditional story that resonates with you and your family. At the end of the story, when the light has returned, the storyteller uses the burning ember to light their candle, and then each candle is lit in turn as the flame is shared from one candle to the next around the circle.

Next, head to the place where you will have the bonfire. Bring your candles and the ember. Use the ember to light the kindling under the Yule log, and send your wishes to heaven.

Now is the time for libations, songs, and gratitude offerings.

*Pairings*

- Book: *Celtic Folklore Cooking* by Joanne Asala—a lovely introduction to Celtic food, culture, and folklore
- Music: "The Mummer's Dance" by Loreena McKennitt
- Resource: Sacred Living Movement Year Planner, brought to you by Sacred Living Movement UK—a yearly planner full of recipes, seasonal inspiration, and crafting

# Journal

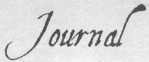

What are your plans for the year ahead? How are you welcoming the light into all aspects of your life?

_____

_____

_____

_____

_____

_____

_____

_____

_____

_____

_____

_____

_____

_____

_____

_____

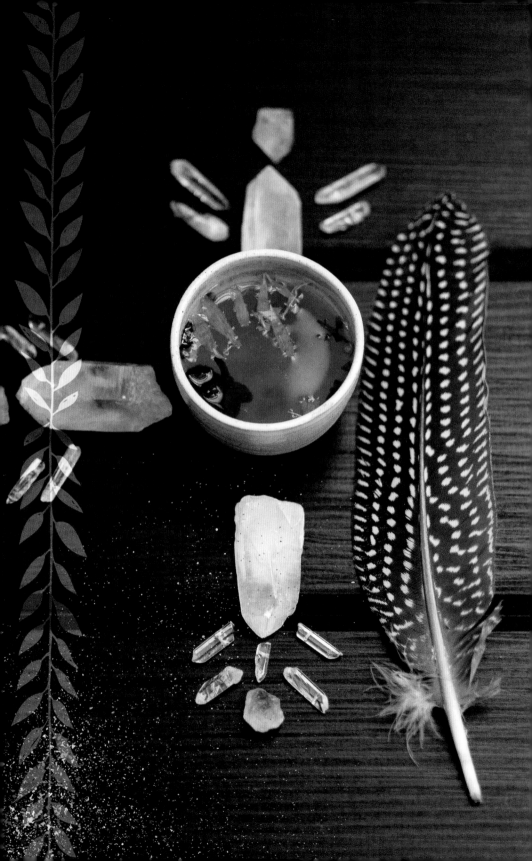

*the seed*

chapter 31

You are connected to the life-force energy of the universe. This powerful current runs through every cell, inside and outside of you. It pulses from your heart to the core of the planet, and rings through to the celestial bodies above you. From the harmony of spheres to the dance of the planets and stars, to the fluttering of leaves in the wind, everything is resonating with this life-force energy. You are a body in motion, even when you are still and silent.

As you enter the closing seasons of your life, time and energy are precious. Your body wisely begins to conserve your vital force for the grace of your longevity. There is a great mystery to these years of transition. The sacred secret of the seed is that it is both the last transformation of the plant and the first. It contains all the knowledge and wisdom of the vast universe, uniquely crafted by the most recent growing seasons, and holds the full potential for rebirth.

## FAMILY WELLNESS: *Bone Health*

Your bones, while strong and solid, are changing shape all the time. You continually make new bone, and old bone material gets reabsorbed into the body. Bones comprise your internal structure, and protect your tender internal organs. In fact, your bones are shaped by your regular activities. Skeletons discovered in ancient burial sites show this shaping—the bodies of archers, for instance, are identified by their one-sided enlarged scapula, where the shoulder blade grew bigger due to the repeated pulling of the bowstring. As you age, your bones grow and absorb less efficiently; over the age of thirty, we create less bone mass. However, there are ways to reduce bone loss:[83]

- **Make sure you are getting your minerals.** Bones need minerals, especially calcium and magnesium. Eat mineral-rich foods such as broth, almonds, oily fish, and kale.

- **Maintain a good uptake of vitamin D.** Good sources include sunshine, oily fish, and eggs.

- **Weight-bearing exercises** such as walking, kettlebell, or dancing help drive calcium into the bones. They also help you grow strong bones in general. Be sure to check with your care provider before starting any fitness regimen.

## SPIRITUAL APPLICATION: *Becoming a Wise One*

As you cycle through different life stages, you gain real practical experience. You learn the power of honoring your soul path and your heart wisdom. Carrying and passing down this awareness for the next generation is a real gift. Maintaining the hard-won path of a higher soul vibration for those behind you, and tending it with care, are the tasks of a spiritual warrior. Your greatest tools for this duty are the skills of empathy, patience, humor, and trust.

## SOUL CHALLENGE: *Elder*

Affirm your knowledge and life experiences. Sit with a piece of paper titled, "I Know This …" Write quickly, without overthinking. Explore and validate your life journey. Know that this wisdom is worthy to be shared and honored.

## GLOBAL APOTHECARY: *Crystal Grids*

Crystals are the bones of the Earth. They hold memory, and provide structure and connection to the flow of source energy. Using a grid can amplify and intensify the innate energetic force of the crystals. Grids increase the harmony of crystals with their environment and with your focused intentions.

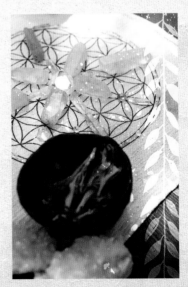

Grids are usually made using sacred geometric patterns—you can draw these yourself on plain cloth, or buy them ready-to-use. This is an opportunity to imbue your clear intention into every layer of the craft. Popular designs include the Golden Spiral, the Flower of Life, and the Star, but you need not be limited to these. Ask your crystal—chances are that they will have a helpful suggestion for you to intuit.

Grids are commonly made up of one center crystal with a radiating pattern of small crystals marking out the shape of the grid. Each stone is charged with your clear intention. There are no rules about how to choose these crystals. Some people use a pendulum, while others use their intuition. Much of this work is done with subtle feelings, so do not overthink it; be clear and light with your heart. Choose small crystals, and place them on your design around one focal crystal in the center. Ask each crystal to support you in your greater intention.

The last step is to activate the grid. Take a crystal point (also called a wand), and sit quietly for a few minutes. Center yourself with your breath and come into the present moment. Use the point to connect the crystals energetically, drawing a line from the center, first pausing to really feel the energy flowing from the universe through your body and the crystal point, and deep into the grid's center crystal. Then repeat this, moving from stone to stone, connecting them all. This is all about practicing your clear focus and pure intention. Once you have finished, step back and feel the vibrations of the grid.

There is no set amount of time to leave the grid activated with your crystals. Keep feeling into the energy, and make sure to give your grid the proper TLC when you think it needs it.

## Conjuring and Crafting

### ANCESTOR-HONORING ALTAR

If you look deeply into the palm of your hand, you will see your parents and all the generations of your ancestors. All of them are alive in this moment because each is present in your body;

you are the continuation of each of these people. (Thanks to Thich Nhat Hanh for this thought.)

Opening yourself to ancient knowledge allows you to tap your personal legacy in the world. Looking to the past allows you to plant seeds for your future, and helps to unfold your soul's purpose in the world. Spend some time researching your family tree, learning where your clan is from and what they did in the world. Remember that their wisdom lives in your bones, and in the bones of your children. Open that book of knowledge with pride, and use this heritage to specially honor your ancestors.

This dark season is a sacred time of year when the veil between the worlds is thin. Your honoring altar may include close family members, or inspiring folks from the past who have lifted you in ways that they could never know. The human experience is one of struggle and inspiration, dark and light, yin and yang, and this is the time to say "thank you" to those who have inspired you in so many ways.

Create a space in your home to host pictures of ancestors who have crossed over the veil, and add candles, flowers, bones, and maybe favorite artifacts or talismans that represent each person. Invite your community or family to be a part of building this altar, and add something for the ancestors of others as well.

---

## VITALITY TONIC

*Shared with us by the wonderful herbalist Sarah Josey from Golden Poppy Herbal Apothecary.*

Perfect for both men and women, this herbal tonic is great for restoring vigor.

- Large Mason jar
- Cheesecloth

- Storage bottle
- Large pot
- About 14 ounces water
- ¼ ounce *muira puama* bark
- ¼ ounce *he shou wu* (*Fallopia multiflora*, or Chinese knotweed) dried leaf
- ¼ ounce nettle leaf
- ¼ ounce dried alfalfa leaf
- ¼ ounce *Tribulus terrestris* (also known as *bindii*, caltrop, or puncture vine)
- About 10 ounces brandy (enough to cover the herbs)
- ¼ ounce maca powder
- ¼ ounce cocoa powder
- ¼ teaspoon vanilla extract
- Honey, to sweeten

In a large Mason jar, place all the herbs except the maca and cocoa powder, and shake well to mix. Pour enough brandy over the herbs to cover them by one inch above the herbs. After the first few days you may need to add more brandy as the herbs soak up some of it up, which is okay.

Seal and label the jar, and place it out of the sun. Shake it daily for two weeks, each time thinking of nothing but vitality, youth, and vigor. At the end of two weeks, strain through the cheesecloth, squeezing as much brandy as possible out of the herbs; reserve the liquid for later.

Place the herbs into a large pot, and just cover them with water (about 14 ounces). Simmer with the lid on until the water is reduced by half. Strain out the herbs through the cheesecloth, being sure to squeeze as much liquid out as possible. Compost the herbs.

To the warm herbal tea water, add the infused brandy, maca powder, cocoa powder, and vanilla extract. Stir to combine. Stir in honey to sweeten it to your liking.

Place in a bottle and label it.

As desired, take 1 teaspoon–1 Tablespoon daily. Be sure to shake well before each use, to mix up the powders. **Note:** Maca and *Tribulus* both have known hormone-modulating effects, so if you are on HRT please discuss their use with your care provider before consuming this tonic.

Add energetic potency to this tonic by mixing it into a cup of Marigold Tea (Chapter 27) and charging it with a crystal grid and your blessings before drinking.

## Pairings

- Tool: Crystal grid cloth—You can purchase cloths with sacred geometry patterns already printed on them. Etsy is a great place to look online for these.

- Class: Sacred Wise Woman from the Sacred Living Movement. Step into your wise years with humor, reverence, grace, and honoring, in the circle of sisterhood.

# Journal

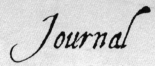

Use this space to explore your connection to the cycles of life: Where are you now? How do you feel about moving through each stage?

_____

_____

_____

_____

_____

_____

_____

_____

_____

_____

_____

_____

_____

_____

_____

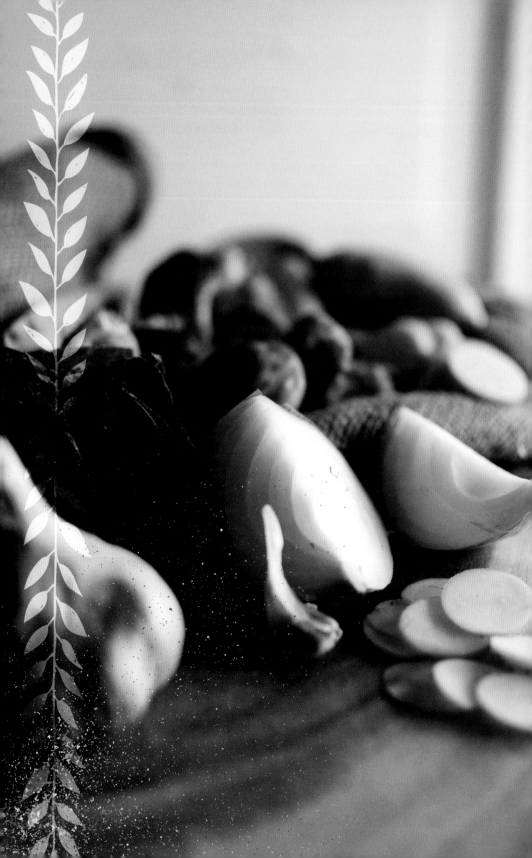

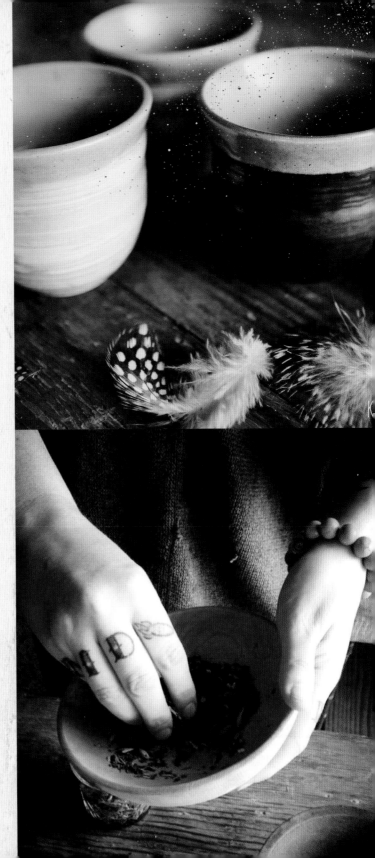

# nourish

*you are what you eat*

---

**chapter 32**

*Nourishment is sustenance that feeds the whole of who you are. Having a bounty of work does not always equate to happiness or health; exquisite foods may pass your lips, and you may still have hunger; material offerings may keep you warm, yet your heart may still be set in yearning, if you do not know love. Nourishment is a language that speaks to of all parts of you. It is the fuel for your cells, your heart, and your spirit. Consider now how you feed yourself—in every way.*

## FAMILY WELLNESS: *Fever 101*

Fever is a vital defense of the body. It is a high temperature, usually over the normal range of 98–100° F, that helps to fight bacterial and viral conditions. The heat increases the mobility and activity of white blood cells, both of which are key functions in immune response.

While fevers play an important role in fighting illness, very high fevers in children can be dangerous and scary. When in doubt, please contact your care provider. Always trust your parenting instincts—you know your child better than anyone, and you know when something is off or different in your child. Do not be worried about asking for support or investigating health concerns. No question is too small when it comes to the health of yourself and your loved ones.

### Gentle ways to nourish when there is fever

With mild fevers, it may be best to wait it out. In these cases, comfort measures are best. These include a cool, damp cloth on the forehead, loose clothing, and adequate hydration.

A Cochrane systematic review found studies demonstrating that tepid sponging alone helps to reduce fever in children as effectively as antipyretic medicines.[84, 85] Tepid sponging is done with water about the same temperature as the skin—not too hot or too cold. Overcooling can force the body to work harder when it is already under stress.

## SPIRITUAL APPLICATION: *Feeding All Parts of You*

You are a complex and fascinating soul. What stimulates your mind and stirs your heart is unique to you. When you are caught up in the flow of daily life, it is easy to forget to water your dreams and feed your thoughts. Trying new activities that push you beyond your comfortable routine might awaken long-dormant parts of you. Or perhaps what you really need is a good book and some time off, to rouse the flames of imagination that have burned low. Maybe your inner teenager wants to have a night out on the town, or maybe your inner child wants to watch clouds go by. Know you are worthy of love, and take some time to nourish these parts of you that may have been left untended.

## SOUL CHALLENGE: *Spirit Food*

How do you feed your soul? Is it listening to the ocean, being in the woods, singing in the car, or dancing under the stars? Choose a couple of daily practices that feed your soul, and spend five or ten minutes doing them, every day for a week.

## GLOBAL APOTHECARY: *Salt Sock for Earaches*

Salt socks are wonderfully soothing for the pain of earaches. They do not treat the underlying issue, however, so be sure to check in with your care provider, especially if the pain is recurring or accompanied by a fever.

Pour 2 cups of rock salt into a white, 100%-cotton sock, and tie or sew it closed. Heat in a dry pan on the stovetop, turning every minute or so until warmed through. Do not leave unattended! Once warm, place on sore ear—very comforting!

# *Conjuring and Crafting*

---

## BONE BROTH

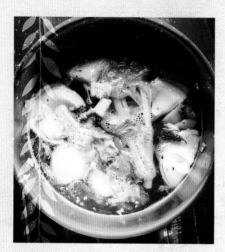

Broths provide essential minerals and nutrients. They are easy on the digestive system, and promote overall health. There is nothing quite like a simple broth to restore body, mind, and soul. These recipes will help keep the inner fires burning.

The easiest way we have found to make bone broth is in a slow-cooker. We often roast a whole chicken. Then we strip the meat from the carcass, and cut up the bones to let the marrow out—poultry scissors make the job very easy.

- Large crockpot or stock pot
- Chicken or other bones (chicken feet are also great for getting more gelatin into the broth)
- 2–4 carrots
- 2–4 ribs of celery
- 2–4 onions, skin and all
- 1–2 heads of garlic, peels and all
- Optional—ginger, lemongrass, chili, galangal, turmeric, parsley (use with caution if breastfeeding, as it can reduce milk supply), peppercorns, dill, sage, or rosemary
- Water, to cover
- 4 Tablespoons apple cider vinegar
- Salt, to taste

If not already cooked, roast your bones in the oven at about 400° F for about 20 minutes, to bring out the flavor and start the cooking process.

Put bones in the pot, and cover them with water. Add apple cider vinegar—this helps release the minerals from the bones. Then add vegetables and bring to a boil, skimming off any foam. Once boiling, turn down and allow to simmer for 24 hours for chicken or fish bones, and around 48 hours for beef, lamb, or pork bones. You know it is ready when the bones are soft and begin to crumble. Strain the bones and cooked vegetables from the broth.

You can drink this broth as-is, or incorporate it into your favorite recipes such as risotto, soup, stir-fries, rice, and noodles. This broth freezes well, and stores well in the refrigerator.

## POTASSIUM BROTH

Potassium broth is a vegan version of Bone Broth, and is also packed with minerals. It's inexpensive and easy to make.

- Large crockpot or stock pot
- 2–4 ribs of celery
- 3–4 potatoes, skin and all
- 2–4 onions, skin and all
- 3 carrots
- 2 yellow beets
- 1–2 heads of garlic, skin and all
- Thumb-size piece of fresh turmeric
- Thumb-size piece of fresh garlic
- 5–8 shiitake mushrooms
- 1 piece of kombu seaweed
- 5–7 black peppercorns

- 1 bunch of parsley (If breastfeeding, you may want to avoid parsley, as it can reduce milk supply.)
- 1 bunch or cilantro
- Salt, to taste

Add everything to your pot except the parsley and cilantro. Cover with water. Bring to a boil and simmer for a couple of hours. Add parsley and cilantro, and simmer for another hour. Strain all the vegetables from your broth, and gift them to your compost. Adjust seasoning to taste.

You can drink this broth as-is, or incorporate it into your favorite recipes such as risotto, soup, stir-fries, rice, and noodles. It also freezes well, and stores well in the refrigerator.

---

## COOL MIST

A special fairy mister to soothe fevers.

- 3-ounce spritzer bottle
- 2½ ounces pure water
- 10 drops sandalwood essential oil
- 10 drops rose essential oil
- 10 drops lavender essential oil (for under age six; for age six-plus, use peppermint)
- ½ ounce witch hazel
- 3 drops silver gem essence
- 3 drops white lotus or gardenia flower essence

Mix the essential oils and the witch hazel together. Add to the water. Mix in the flower and gem essences, and pour into spritzer bottle.

Spritz as needed to bring cooling and comfort.

*Pairings*

- Food: Mineral-rich salt such as pink Himalayan or the Maldon or Real Salt brands of sea salt—these contain trace minerals not found in regular table salt.

- Book: *Nourished Kitchen* by Jennifer McGruther—a traditional-food cookbook to inspire you in the kitchen.

- Resource: *Mother's Wisdom Deck* by Niki Dewart and Elizabeth Marglin. This book and oracle-card deck offer insight and spiritual nourishment, with thoughtful prompts and beautiful artwork.

# Journal

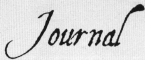

What are your comfort foods? Make a list here.

_____

_____

_____

_____

_____

_____

_____

_____

_____

_____

_____

_____

_____

_____

_____

_____

_____

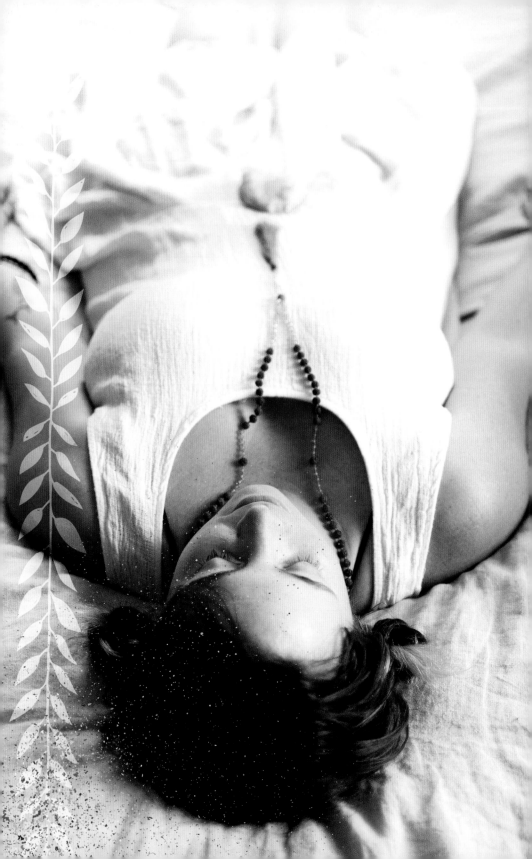

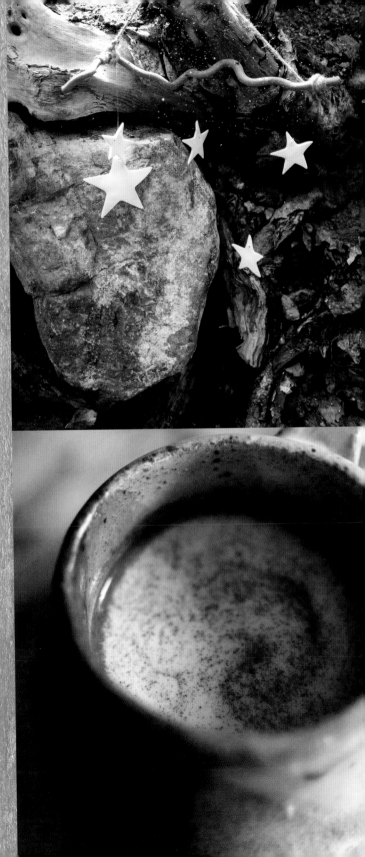

_rest_

_the deep drink_

chapter 33

What are your own food traditions, handed down by your family? What feeds your soul?

*Drop in, slow down, and coil inward. Deliciously restorative when intentional, rest calls to your every cell for ultimate replenishment. You know in your bones the peace of the winter quiet. You appreciate the transcendent silence of the bejeweled night sky, and the calm fortitude of the snowy forest. This moment is the pause after the exhalation—that tranquil bliss where everything just stops. Curl into your coziest spaces, and get ready to recharge your inner fires.*

## FAMILY WELLNESS: *Sleep*

So often, sleep is undervalued as a key factor in health and wellness. But giving your body the time to rest supports optimal health. Did you know that during sleep your cerebrospinal fluid is flushed of toxins? Sleep has also has been shown to improve learning and longevity, reduce stress, and balance hormones and weight, in addition to enhancing mental health.[86]

A great way to explore the quality of your sleep as a family is to keep a sleep journal for a week. Here are some questions to explore:

· How do you feel when you wake in the morning—well rested, or do you want to sleep longer?

· How many hours of sleep do you get every night?

· What is normal for you?

· How do you sleep—are you a light sleeper and up many times in the night?

· Do you wake around the same time every day?

· Do you go to sleep around the same time every night?

Good sleep practices include staying hydrated, turning off all electronic screens well before bedtime, and sleeping in a dark room.

If you feel you may have sleep issues, talk to your care provider about getting a sleep assessment.

## SPIRITUAL APPLICATION: *Hitting the Pause Button*

We believe that if you give your body the right tools and enough time, you can heal from anything. Hitting the pause button allows you to step away from a hard situation or personal struggle. It is a potent tool for regrouping, restoring, and resting—spiritually and emotionally as well as physically. Creating this kind of space gives you time to process and check in with your heart.

## SOUL CHALLENGE: *Pause and Reflect*

Next time you are in a heated, volatile, or painful situation, hit the pause button. Set a clear boundary for time away from the strife—maybe thirty minutes, or even overnight. Charge yourself with the task of emotionally leaving that situation so that you can truly reintegrate your feelings, meditate, and respond from your highest self. Perhaps go outside, take a deep breath, and do not make any decisions. You could process your feelings through journaling if you need to, sifting through them at a slow and thoughtful pace. When the time is up, come back to the situation with a fresh outlook and distilled thoughts.

## GLOBAL APOTHECARY: *Yoga Nidra*

*Yoga nidra* means "yogic sleep," and is essentially a deep state of relaxation. It is one of the deepest levels of relaxation while still conscious. There are lots of free resources around to help you try this practice, including the Yoga Nidra Network, which describes the practice as "an opportunity to re-encounter the essential truth of who you really are."[87]

# Conjuring and Crafting

Tranquil, restful conjuring for the still winter nights.

---

## SWEET-SLEEP BATH SOAK

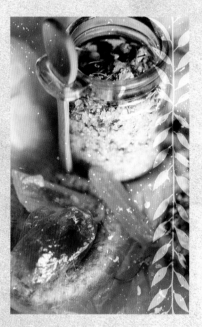

The Epsom salts in this mixture contain magnesium, which helps soothe muscles and promote sleep.

- ½ pound Epsom salts
- 1 cup dried, powdered rose petals
- 1 cup dried, powdered chamomile blossoms
- 1 cup dried, powdered lavender blossoms
- 1 cup dried, powdered lemon balm leaves
- 7 drops thyme flower essence

Mix everything together and store in a large jar. Use about ½–1 cup per bath.

---

## DREAM MILK

*Radha Schwaller has shared this nourishing and calming bedtime milk recipe.*

Spiced warm milk (almond, rice, goat, or cow) is deeply grounding and balancing to *vata,* which is the predominant energy of an active mind. Next time you can't sleep, or just want to relax deeply before bed, try this recipe.

- 1 cup raw whole milk or almond milk

- I pinch cinnamon
- I pinch nutmeg
- I pinch powdered rose petals
- I pinch ground cardamom
- I pinch ground clove

Put everything in a pan, and simmer gently for about 5–10 minutes, until warmed through—no need to boil it.

Sip thoughtfully. Here's to your bliss-filled sweet dreams tonight!

## Pairings

- Supplement: Magnesium—a key mineral in hydration, it is essential for melatonin regulation, and relaxes the nervous system.

- Crystal: Moonstone—said to be the tears of an ancient moon goddess, this crystal is wonderful to aid in connection with the moon. Place it under your pillow, keep it in your Sacred Space, or perhaps wear it as a *mala* (bead necklace).

- Flower Essence: Thyme flower essence—quiet and still, this essence spools your dispersed energy gently back into your body.

# Journal

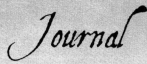

Use this space to track your sleep for the next week.

_____

_____

_____

_____

_____

_____

_____

_____

_____

_____

_____

_____

_____

_____

_____

_____

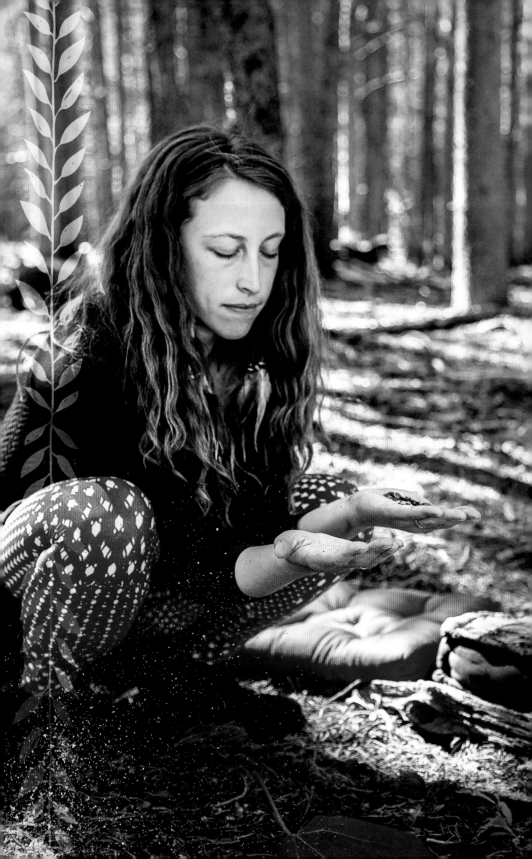

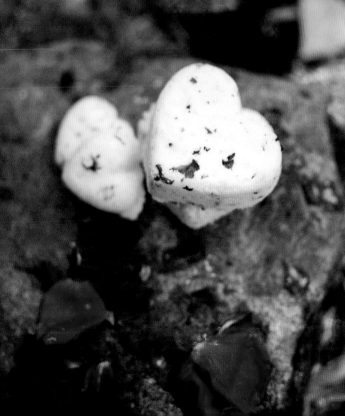

# gratitude

## the path of enlightenment

chapter 34

*The world around you is full of the most wondrous and precious mysteries. Being in communion with these adds depth to the quality of your life, in both your physical and spiritual realities. Do you know the beauty of a hummingbird in flight? Does your heart sigh with childlike awe at the blossoming of a flower? Do you notice the way the light of a sunset paints the sky? Noticing beauty, and being in gratitude for all that you witness, infuses your heart with a tangible warmth that spills over to color each new day with promise.*

## FAMILY WELLNESS: *Gratitude is Medicine*

Scientists have recently begun to research the benefits of a daily gratitude practice. Living in abundance begins and ends with gratitude. Not only does this way of living help you see the blessings you have, it impacts your well-being in several ways. Some benefits include:[88]

- Stronger immune systems and lower blood pressure
- Higher levels of positive emotions
- More joy, optimism, and happiness
- Acting with more generosity and compassion
- Feeling less lonely and isolated

### *Practical ways to play with gratitude*

- **Keep a daily gratitude-practice pinboard,** with notes and affirmations.
- **Make a game of noticing new things each day.** You know you are grateful for the roof over your head, for example. Push yourself—what else can you find?
- **Find people and their actions to be grateful for,** instead of focusing on material things.
- **Send a message to someone who has helped you,** and notice how this makes you feel.
- **Make gratitude a dinnertime practice for the whole family,** and inspire each other.

## SPIRITUAL APPLICATION: *A Spiritual Lifeline*

Gratitude can be work, especially when life is compressed with various challenges—but those are the moments when the practice is most vital. It can be a spiritual lifeline when hope is lost.

If you can find anything, no matter how small, to be grateful for in the darkest of times, it can be the first step toward something better and, even more importantly, toward spiritual mastery. One of my favorite Buddhist quotes is, "Meditate for twenty minutes everyday. If you cannot find twenty minutes, meditate for an hour." Making the time for gratitude will serve your highest good in ways that will give you tangible results.

Sometimes the simplest place to start is by being grateful for the miracle of life. You are alive, right now in this moment, and you could choose to be grateful for your breath and the beat of your heart. Pushing this further, can you find a way to be grateful for something difficult that has happened in your life? Soul-stretching to look at life lessons and challenges in this way opens your heart, and breathes light into the shadowy corners.

## SOUL CHALLENGE: *Gratitude*

This particular practice may be a real soul-stretch for you, but the work is liberating like no other. Choose a situation in your life where someone has wronged you—can you find a way to be grateful about it, or some aspect of it? Write that person a letter of gratitude for the lessons you were gifted from this situation.

## GLOBAL APOTHECARY: *Barefoot Breathing*

Here is a simple practice to foster your connection with nature. "Barefoot breathing" is the practice of touching your bare feet to the earth and—well, breathing. Such a simple activity can have many benefits, including discharging electromagnetic energies and rebalancing our internal magnetic and emotional poles. It is especially wonderful if you have been sitting at a computer a lot, or around Wi-Fi, cell phones, and modern life in general. This is a very grounding practice.

It best done in the morning while the fresh dew is blanketing the earth. But it is perfectly okay to do this anytime of day.

## How to do "barefoot breathing"

Step outside with your bare feet touching the earth. You need to have contact with the actual earth, so no standing on pavement, sidewalks, or driveways.

Once your feet have contacted the earth, stand relaxed with your spine straight and a slight bend in your knees. Your spine is relaxed and open. Imagine the top of your head connected to the sky by a golden cord that allows your body to gently dangle. Your feet are supported by the Earth with a strong and steady lift that pushes back against your soles.

Allow yourself to feel a grounding cord that stretches from your tailbone into the center of the Earth. You are connected and stable. Here you are, perfectly centered between heaven and Earth—a bright, loving soul in a human body.

Now just breathe. Allow Mother Earth to take any unwanted energy from you. She is the ultimate recycler, and will take what you give her, clean it, and use it somewhere else. With each breath in, you are more centered and more connected. With each breath out, you let go of excess energy, emotion, or low-vibration thoughts. It is

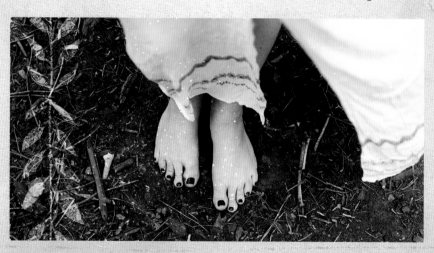

all energy—just release it. There is no judgment, no attachment, and no doubt in this journey. You are simply making space for what is new and fresh to be activated within your being.

Enjoy three more rounds of this breathing practice, and thank the Earth and the sky for their plentiful gifts of abundance.

When you are ready, allow your breath to soften back to your own rhythm. You are filled with light, and connected to heaven and Earth—a shining, refreshed spirit in your human body.

## Conjuring and Crafting

### GRATITUDE TO FAMILY: *Thank-You Stones*

Surprise family members with sweet gratitude notes acknowledging a deed or act of service your loved one has done, or simply saying why you love that person.

- Pen and paper
- Your powers of observation
- The element of surprise

Use your powers of observation to notice the little things your loved ones have done: Did they pick you up and give you a ride somewhere? Did they give a heart gift? Children often give heart gifts, like picking flowers for you, or sharing a beloved toy with you. Perhaps someone took the time to make you something you like to eat on a regular basis. Look around—you will find something!

Write your loved one a little note thanking them for this service, deed, or gift. Or simply write a love note about how amazing you think they are.

Leave the note in a place where they will find it.

## GRATITUDE TO YOURSELF
## AND YOUR FRIENDS: *Relaxing Fizzy Bath Bombs*

*Sarah Josey from Golden Poppy Herbal Apothecary
has created these lovely bath-bomb recipes for you to create
and maybe gift to your friends.*

- Large mixing bowl
- Mixing spoon
- Bath-bomb molds (find these online, or try using plastic Easter eggs, silicone muffin trays, or anything of similar size)
- Paper towels
- 18 ounces baking soda
- 7 ounces citric acid
- 3 ounces sea salt
- 6 ounces Epsom salt
- 3 ⅕ ounces sweet almond oil
- ⅕ ounce rose petals
- 10 drops lavender essential oil
- 10 drops neroli essential oil
- 10 drops rose essential oil

Be sure your bowl and spoon are completely dry before mixing, as any water will cause the bath bombs to begin to fizz!

Mix the salts, baking soda, and citric acid together in a bowl. Sprinkle in the rose petals. (You can also add other flowers, such as lavender or calendula, for more color and beauty.) Add the almond oil, and drop in the essential oils. Mix well. Press the mix into the molds, being sure to pack them as tightly as possible. If using a muffin tray, place a large, heavy book on top of the filled molds to weight them down. After about 20 minutes, remove the bombs from the molds or tins and lay the bombs on the paper towels to dry overnight.

Store in a moisture-proof container, and add one to a fully filled bath for your enjoyment!

## Pairings

- Book: *Peace is Every Step* by Thich Nhat Hanh—a powerful, beautiful, and wise book on mindfulness and gratitude.
- Movement: Pay It Forward, based on the book by Catherine Ryan Hyde, aims to create a ripple effect of good deeds through acts of kindness "paid forward" from one person to another.

# *Journal*

Start your gratitude practice here. List five
things every day that you are grateful for.

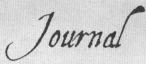

_____

_____

_____

_____

_____

_____

_____

_____

_____

_____

_____

_____

_____

_____

_____

_____

_____

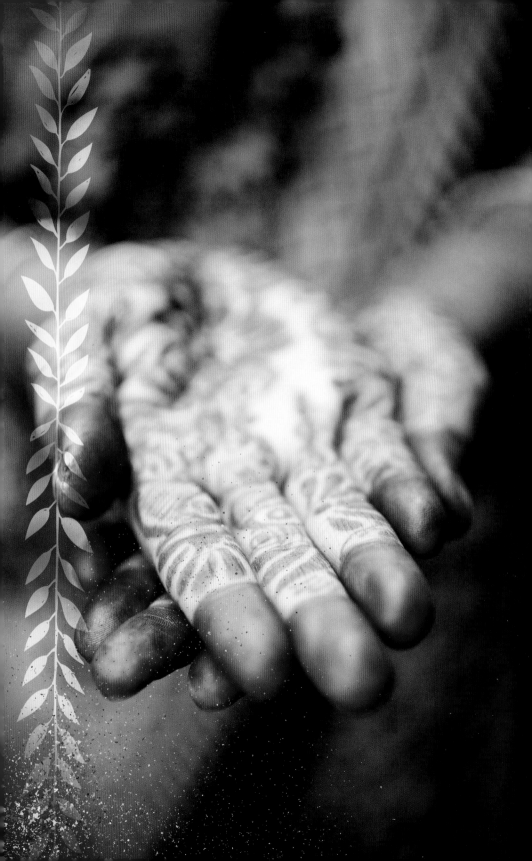

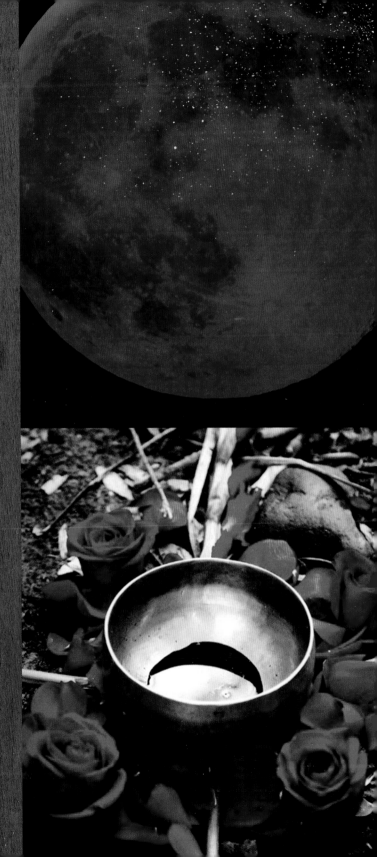

*what the moon sees*

# the moon

## chapter 35

*The moon keeps time with the rhythm of the cosmos, and this monthly metronome infuses your very* DNA. *You are inextricably linked to the waxing and waning tides, even if it feels mysterious and hidden. The soft luminous light of the moon has the power to brighten shadowy corners, and influence physical and emotional waters. This is the light that reveals hidden truths—your secret wisdom and deep understanding awaits. Moonlight is responsive, receptive, and revealing, and if you reach your hands up in timeless salutation, her glow will cascade enormous blessings over every part of you.*

## FAMILY WELLNESS: *Menstrual Health*

The monthly cycle of menstruation and the monthly procession of the moon are a dance between your earthly body and the body of the heavens. Some women ovulate with the energy of the full moon, and bleed with the new. Others ovulate with the new moon and bleed with the full.

If your cycle doesn't regulate with that obvious rhythm, looking at where the moon is in your birth chart may offer a clue. For example, with a moon in Pisces on your natal chart, you may find yourself bleeding when the moon is in Pisces, no matter what her phase. Or the moon phase from your natal chart may be affecting you—if the moon was a waxing gibbous on the day of your birth, you may find that you cycle with that particular phase. But this is just another way to flow, and none of these is the definitive way everyone's body must work.

The monthly cycle is a mini-walk through the energetic seasons of the year, mirrored by the moon's changing energy through the month. When you ovulate, it is like spring, representing the Wood element in Chinese medicine—your eggs burst forth, and you have momentum and action. Then you have the sultry Fire-element power of summer—the hot and sexy time of desire and expansive connection. The egg either gets fertilized and attaches to the wall of the uterus to ripen, or you ripen energetically, potent and waiting for the opportunity to express this potential. The ripening phase corresponds to the Earth element, or harvest time in the cycle of the year. Then you move into the Metal or Air phase, as in late autumn—the shedding and releasing of your bleeding days. These days are slower, and energetically lower. It is a time for reflection and refinement. Then, as the bleeding finishes, you have the moment of the void—the Water element, the winter stillness where anything is possible.

The five-element cycle can be used to describe your journey through womanhood as well. You begin in winter, the Water element season—the time of the ovum, all possibility and mystery. Then you enter spring, the place of Wood element's wild growth, and mature from childhood into puberty. At puberty, you become active and sensual; the Fire power of summer awakens within you. Then you mature into the Earth-element quality of your ripe years, where you are fertile in mind and body, experienced enough to allow the fruits of your life to mellow and ripen. Next you enter the time of refinement, the letting-go, the transition of the autumnal Metal/Air phase when your cycle begins to end.

Your menstruation cycle ends because your body is wise, and knows when it is time to conserve your energy for longevity. You return to winter, your place of deep knowledge and quiet strength. Once the body has had time to rest and process, you move again into spring, renewed and reformed; you continue to experience these energetic cycles—and the procession of the spiral continues.

The process of making blood and losing blood each month takes a lot of energy. Here are a few of our favorite tips for optimal menstrual health:

- **Take time out during bleeding days.** Many cultures see bleeding days as a time when women are especially powerful and spiritually open. They give women space to work creatively with this special power during this time every month. During your monthly moon, you are accessing your place of deep power and inner knowing, and need sacred time to tap your artistic brilliance.

- **Food is medicine,** and it is the best preventative medicine around. This means avoiding known endocrine-system disruptors found in processed foods, conventional wheat products, refined sugar, or large amounts of caffeine and dairy.

- **Ditch the toxins!** Consider using sustainable hygiene products such as a menstrual cup, reusable pads, or even biodegradable, organic disposables to catch your blood every month. Super-toxic, ultra-absorbent, fragranced products may cause problems with vaginal irritation. Changing to reusable products is kinder to both your body and Mama Earth.

- **Look after your adrenals!** Stress, overwork, over-exercise, lack of sleep, caffeine, alcohol, and sugar all take a heavy toll on your adrenal glands and endocrine (hormone) system. Of course, nothing can replace a good night's sleep!

- **Get moving!** Your monthly flow wants to flow free. Your energy needs movement. Heavy cramping in Traditional Chinese Medicine is a sign that something is energetically stagnant or stuck—physically or emotionally trapped. Moving outside in nature, even just going for a short walk, will get things moving. Yoga and dance are also great movement activities that can motivate your highest self.

- **Annual liver cleanse**: This is best done in spring, around the equinox, and is not recommended if you are pregnant or breast-feeding. Be sure to work with a trained practitioner—it will make the liver cleanse easy and simple. Liver cleanses usually involve herbs and foods that help break down fats and toxins stored in the liver, and cleanse them from your body for good. A well-functioning liver is a key to smooth menstrual flow.

- **Body work and/or acupuncture**: Ayurvedic massage, Mayan abdominal massage, shiatsu, reflexology, acupuncture, and kinesiology—just to name a few—are all healing modalities that can help you maintain a healthy cycle every month.

## SPIRITUAL APPLICATION: *The Shadow*

The power of moonlight is to reveal what is hidden; sometimes this is called the "shadow." It is a part of your nature that you may have trouble seeing or accepting. Why is it important to explore these tender and challenging places? Seeing your shadow as part of you helps you integrate all parts of yourself; this is essential for wholeness.

This practice is done without judgment, without the harsh inner voice. It is about witnessing your own humanity—the good, the struggles, the mundane, the bitter, and the gracious—all of it. No one exists without a shadow. When you can model love, forgiveness, and acceptance in yourself, then you can truly offer them to others in your life.

The purpose of exploring your shadow is not to get rid of it, but to learn how to integrate it into your life in a healthy way. When you are open to it, this journey of exploration can be a playful, curious activity of self-discovery.

## SOUL CHALLENGE: *Claim Your Shadow*

Prepare for this soul challenge by writing down a list of your best traits. You can even ask close friends and family members to give you three words that represent you. Then set aside some time to meditate. Turn off all the lights, sit in front of a mirror, and light a candle. Look into your eyes and really see all of you. Out loud, claim your shadow aspects and characteristics by declaring the times you were petty, afraid, tired, angry—all of it. Now smile, and welcome and integrate your whole self by reading to yourself your list of best traits and words. You are all of these. You are whole.

## GLOBAL APOTHECARY: *Moon Magick*

Moon magick is the practice of using the phases of the moon to influence your actions and intentions. Working with the timing of the moon has been done across many cultures for tasks from the planting of seeds and harvesting of food to acting as a conception oracle.

As a general rule, the new moon is best for beginnings; it is the start of the moon's cycle, so it is a great time to manifest new things you need in your life. The full moon adds potency and illumination, and is considered the peak of the cycle. Finally, the dark moon is for releasing and banishing that which does not belong anymore or is not needed.

## Conjuring and Crafting

These recipes support you as you flow through your monthly moon.

---

### LAVENDER AND ROSE COMFORT PILLOW

Create a soothing pillow that can be warmed and used as a compress on tender womb spaces.

- ¾ pound dried lavender buds
- ¼ pound dried rose petals
- Thread and needle, or sewing machine
- Two 16" squares of fabric—your choice of velvet, cotton, brocade, or linen

Sew 3½ sides of the squares together, with the fabric inside-out. Turn the fabric right-side-out and fill the pillow loosely with lavender. Hand-stitch the opening closed, or use a ribbon to tie it off.

Use the pillow on your belly during your moon time, and add a hot-water bottle to enhance the effect.

---

### YONI STEAM

Vaginal steams are a wonderful way to maintain a healthy *yoni* (female genital area). Many cultures have some version of this;

it is most commonly seen in South American and Asian traditions. You do not need to go anywhere to have a vaginal steam, because it is easy to do right in your own home. The purpose of the steam is to nourish the uterus, introduce heat, and support the self-cleaning mechanisms already in action.

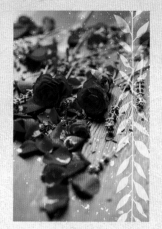

**Note**: Steaming is not recommended for people with an Intrauterine Device (IUD), infection, inflammation, or fever. It is also not recommended during very heavy periods or pregnancy.

1. First, choose your herbs. Some popular herbs include oregano, rosemary, motherwort, calendula, and yarrow. It is lovely to add some aromatics such as rose or lavender to your mixture. You want about 1 ounce of dried plant material, or 2 ounces if fresh. **Note:** Do not use essential oils in liquid form for vaginal steams, as they are too concentrated and volatile for this purpose.

2. Put the herbs in a pot, cover them with about 2 quarts of water, and simmer for about 15 minutes. Turn off the heat, and let steep another 5 minutes or so. You can also use a slow-cooker, which works great if you are using a steaming stool.

3. Place the pot under a chair with open slits, or a stool specifically designed for this purpose. Some women use the toilet by placing a pot inside it—a large enough bowl or pot with handles fits perfectly.

4. Remove your underwear, and sit over the steaming herbal water with a large blanket wrapped around your waist. Be sure the steam is not too hot! If it is super-hot, pull the pot away for a few minutes and try again until the steam feels comfortable.

5. Make sure there are no cold drafts in the room. Keep well covered in a thick, cozy blanket, and wear socks to maintain a warm body equilibrium.

6. Steam for about 20 minutes. The steam introduces healing heat and plant oils into the uterus, cervix, and ovaries.

7. Afterward, you should ideally keep warm for at least an hour; resting in bed is a great way to do this. Even better, do this right before you go to sleep, to really seal in the benefits.

## Pairings

- Supplement: D-Mannose is a naturally occurring sugar that bonds to *E. coli* bacteria and keeps them from sticking to your intestines and urinary tract. It is a great preventative measure against urinary-tract infections caused by these bacteria.

- Book: *Moon Mysteries* by Nikiah Seeds and Nao Sims—a gorgeous and wise companion for people with menstrual cycles.

- Class: Sacred Blood Mysteries by The Jessicas at the Sacred Living Movement. This is a three-week class that explores the mysteries of menstruation.

# *Journal*

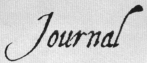

Try tracking your own moon cycle. Keep notes on how you feel during each phase of the moon this month.

_____

_____

_____

_____

_____

_____

_____

_____

_____

_____

_____

_____

_____

_____

_____

_____

_____

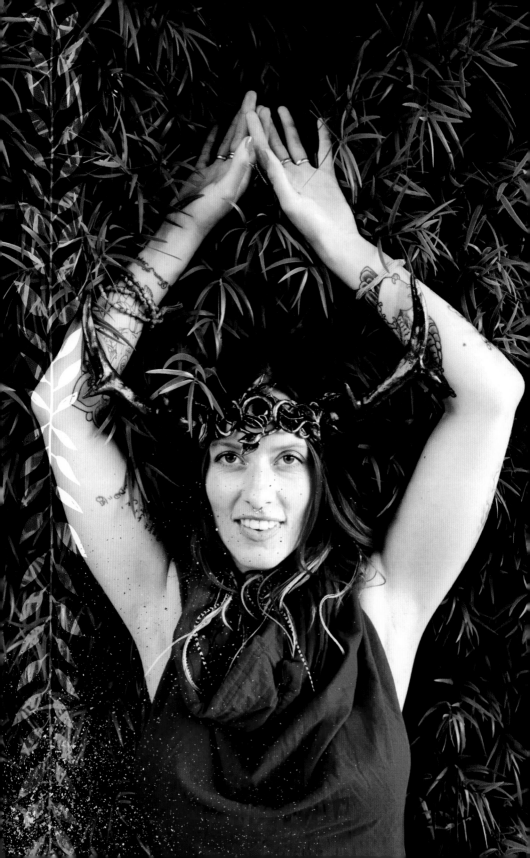

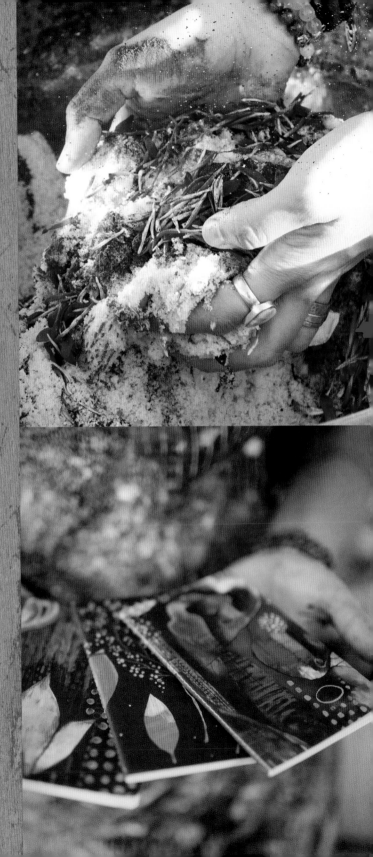

# conjure

## limitless & divine

chapter 36

*Your cupboard is stocked. Your heart is full. Your roots are strong. Some of the most potent healing for you and your loved ones comes from your innate know-ing, or what we call your "heart medicine." As you step into your power as healer of your own life, there is one last question—are you limitless? Being limitless means living with curiosity and hope, and being open to receiving all that the uni-verse has to offer. You are boundless in your dreaming and creating, and it is time to embrace the wide expanse of horizon in front you, and walk your medicine path. You are infinite.*

## FAMILY WELLNESS: *Fear vs. Love*

Sometimes a cataclysmic event sucks the very breath from your lungs and steals the color from your world. It seems as if there was only life before the event, and no hope for your life after it. Once the shock has passed, only navigating the new landscape remains—finding your way slowly, picking through the rubble to see what can be salvaged and what must be built anew. What could you possibly have in your Sacred Cupboard for times like this?

The medicine you have for this isn't stored in a jar or distilled into a tonic. What you have in these moments is the resilience of your own heart, your innate capacity to know love, and to be love. Love is a balm like no other.

Here is the truth: You have this one sacred lifetime in this body, with this soul, this path, and these people. No one is leaving here alive. The fragility of mortality is the perfect reason to temper each precious moment with grace. This awareness helps you dig deeper for those extra dollops of patience and generosity.

This outlook is not meant to sweep up the whole wild and multi-faceted range of human emotion into either fear or love, because of course you are free to feel every single emotion. However, when you do not acknowledge your own truth, or when you judge your emo-tions as inappropriate, you can swiftly move into the vast space of fear. When you lose hope, fear is there to greet you; when you live from a place of lack, fear is there to celebrate. However, these places of fear only harm your soul and derail you from your heart-path.

Take time to listen to your inner knowing, and treat yourself with patience and kindness; these are the gifts and practical tools that will help you through the hard days. Every moment, you get to choose whether to live from fear or love. Always and in all ways, choose love.

## SPIRITUAL APPLICATION: *Miracles*

The spiritual tool of believing in a miracle means, at a core level, staying open to the possibility that you do not know everything. In Zen they call this "Beginner's Mind." When you live from Beginner's Mind, you approach the world open and ready to learn. It's a humble place of understanding that each new day brings opportunity for growth.

Whenever there is a lack of flow in your life—whether creative, physical, or emotional—there is more insight and wisdom to be gained. Maybe you feel like you are doing *everything, when the answer might be to do nothing.* Small miracles happen everyday, but they often sparkle in our lives without much acknowledgement. Breathing, waking up everyday, birthing children, falling in love—all are miracles of living this life.

Human beings tend to want more proof of miracles, however, and usually need to be smacked in the face with a big universal gesture before they truly believe in miracles. Challenge yourself to see past the mundane, and into the miraculous beauty that is all around you, and you will invite more of the big stuff to appear, in spades. Be limitless in your dreams, your possibilities, and your awareness. Then truly anything can happen.

## SOUL CHALLENGE: *You Are a Miracle*

First, focusing on your breath, come into your body. This is the home of your Spirit. Do you know how magical your body is? On a cellular level, you are made of stardust and earth. You carry in your body all

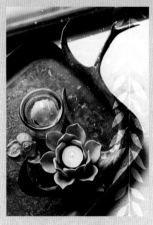

the information from your ancestors—not just human ancestors but your ancestors from all life forms on Planet Earth—animals, plants, and minerals as well as other humans.

Your original cells were carried in your mother's ovaries, which were carried in her mother's ovaries, which were carried in her mother's ovaries, and so on; this unbroken lineage stretches back to the very first woman. You are intimately a part of this cosmos, not separate from it in any way. This is a wonder, a miracle, as is this precious awareness of how magic you truly are. So breathe here, and feel the miracle of life in this body.

Now let go of any preconceived ideas, and enter Beginner's Mind. Remind yourself that you don't know everything, that anything can happen. Each time something challenging comes up this week, choose to enter Beginner's Mind, opening up to the possibility that life is full of limitless potential. Then stand back, and watch the universe collide with your destiny to create perfect miracles right before your eyes!

## GLOBAL APOTHECARY: *Third Eye Chakra—Ajna*

The *ajna* chakra, whose name means "command" or "summoning," opens your intuition, foresight, and imagination. It is located in the center of your forehead, between your eyebrows, which is why it is also called "the third eye." The sound *"sham"* and the color indigo help to open and balance this most creative of chakras.[89]

# *Conjuring and Crafting*

Here is a selection of inspired tools to guide your healing path.

## SALT BOWL CEREMONY

"Going to the bowl" is a completely magical Sacred Living Movement tradition. Instead of doing this in circle with sisterhood, as we do, try it in circle with your family. Salt holds memory, and is an old tool for binding your word with your intentions The old-world tradition is to bind a contract or vow with a pinch of salt in another's satchel; then you could only break your vow if you could take back every grain of salt.

1. Place a selection of flower essences, flowers, dried herbs, spices, crystals, crystal beads, essential oils, and edible glitter in the center of the circle.

2. Fill a large, beautiful bowl with fine sea salt. Place this in the center of the circle as well.

3. Gather your family, and sit around the bowl in a circle. Begin talking about what each of you individually needs right now, and what you need as a family. This is the time to talk about dreams, ask for inspiration, and create hope and possibility. Feel a bubble of energy forming around all of you, full of these pure intentions.

4. When you are ready, each person chooses one or more items from the middle of the circle, to add to the bowl of salt. Go around the circle, and have each person add their ingredient(s) and tell how each ingredient charges the intentions they would like to add into the bowl of pure manifestation. For example, I once sat in circle with a seven-year-old girl who added big, shiny, plastic jewels to the salt bowl, saying that she wished everyone in the world could find their treasure inside themselves. So each person adds their ingredient, and says a wish of what they

want to bring into their life, and why that ingredient will help their intentions fly free into the universe.

5. Each person mixes their ingredient in with their hands until it's well combined.

6. Go around the circle as many times as you want, making sure to get every last wish into the bowl.

7. When you are finished, everyone places one hand in the bowl, and connects with each other through eye contact. Smile, and say together, three times, "As we will it, so shall it be!"

8. Transfer your magic salt into a lovely jar, and add a few pinches to your bath as needed. When you refresh it, keep a spoonful or two to add to the next bowl in order to keep the magic of the sacred bowl flowing.

---

## SACRED MEDICINE ORACLE DECK

Create a homemade divination deck to help you gain deeper insight into your life and energy, and continue your Beginner's Mind learning about the vast mysteries of the universe. Oracle decks offer guidance on using your energy wisely, and bring clarity and divine inspiration into your daily flow.

- 26 blank postcard-size cards
- Pens
- Watercolors
- Paintbrushes
- Glue
- Glitter
- *Washi* (decorated Japanese paper) tape
- Scissors
- Pretty paper and images for collaging
- A box or bag to keep your cards in

Enter your Beginner's Mind, and ask to be guided by your higher self, your spirit allies, and/or your guardian angels. Choose five plants, five animals, five spirit guardians, and five emotions, and decorate each card with these. Create one blank card to give you the option to listen to your wild, untamed heart. Chose an affirmation, poem, or word for each card that will help you connect to the spirit of the card.

Be generous and open with your writing. Write down anything—numbers, colors, animal names, songs, or words. Try not to overthink this; just be in the flow, and write down the messages you receive as you create. Remember that each card will have many meanings, depending on who you are, when you ask the questions, why you are asking them, and what specifically you need to know.

Once you are finished, hold the deck on your hand, close to your heart. Gift the cards a light blow of your breath to infuse them with your *prana,* or life-force. Ask a question in your mind while you shuffle the deck; then pull a card that calls to you. Read the message that you earlier left for yourself, and either meditate on it or journal with it.

As you build your relationship with your cards, you will discover more and more nuanced messages and intuitive understanding.

---

## LIMITLESS ESSENCE

Create an essence to support living from love and understanding your limitless power. Choose a tree, plant, or crystal that calls to your heart. Ask Mother Nature for what you most need, and she will answer.

- Glass bowl
- Piece of cheesecloth, or strainer
- Pint-size Mason jar (to store mother essence)
- I cup pure spring water or sacred water (from a holy or pure source)

- Your nature item to support your limitless living (harvest plant materials when they are alive and at the peak of their growth)
- 1 cup organic vodka or brandy

Follow the "Making a Flower Essence" instructions in Chapter 1.

Take 1 drop on the tongue, or 3 drops diluted in a glass of water and sipped through the day.

## Pairings

- Class: Sacred Medicine Cupboard by the Jessicas at Sacred Living Movement. Take the work of this book deeper with online support and videos.
- Crystal: Citrine—this warm and inviting stone if for calling in energetic abundance, prosperity, and knowing.
- Music: "I Am Light" by India Arie—a thoughtful and moving song that uplifts and infuses you with love.

# *Journal*

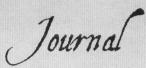

How can you use your Beginner's Mind to refresh your understanding of personal growth, and live in more limitless ways?

_____

_____

_____

_____

_____

_____

_____

_____

_____

_____

_____

_____

_____

_____

_____

_____

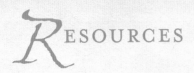

# RESOURCES

The Sacred Living Movement started with a book, a vision, and a dream. Anni Daulter wrote the book *Sacred Pregnancy,* and held a retreat in November 2012 to train visionary birthworkers to "hold space" for birthing mothers, to shift pregnancy and birth from a medicalized experience to something honored and sacred.

After that flagship retreat, the movement grew into more programs and ideas, and has become the grand vision that we now call the Sacred Living Movement. We quickly realized that all aspects of the life journey needed to be addressed, honored, marked, and seen as sacred, so we started developing programs to fit the needs of the communities we were serving.

We have now traveled to over nine different countries, trained nearly 1,000 women to be Sacred Pregnancy Instructors, and expanded who we are and who we want to be by including more classes and retreats that support living a truly Sacred Life. We now offer many live and online trainings to enhance your life and/ or become certified to either teach or offer direct services in your own community. If this movement interests you, please see our list below, and visit our websites.

- Sacred Living Movement (main website): sacredlivingmovement.com
- Sacred Living Movement University: www.sacredlivinguniversity.com
- Sacred Motherhood: www.sacred-motherhood.com
- Sacred Pregnancy: www.sacred-pregnancy.com

- Sacred Postpartum: www.sacredpostpartum.net
- Sacred Beginnings (for mom and baby): www.sacred-beginning.com
- Sacred Relationship (for couples): www.oursacredrelationship.com
- I AM Sisterhood: www.iamsisterhood.com
- Sacred Ayurveda: www.sacred-ayurveda.com
- Sacred Medicine Cupboard: www.sacredmedicinecupboard.com
- Sacred Sweeties (for little girls and their moms): www.sacredsweeties.com
- Sacred Moon Daughters (for girls coming of age): www.sacredmoondaughters.com
- Sacred Menopause: www.sacred-menopause.com
- Sacred Sons: www.sacred-sons.com
- Sacred Brotherhood: https://www.facebook.com/Sacred-Brotherhood-810315092407635/
- Sacred Fertility: www.sacredfertility.com
- Sacred Birth Journey (for pregnant couples): www.sacred-birthjourney.com
- Sacred Midwife: www.sacredmidwife.com
- Sacred Doula: www.sacreddoula.com
- Sacred Milk: www.sacred-milk.com
- Sacred Loss: www.sacred-loss.com
- Sacred Medicine Woman: www.sacred-medicinewoman.com
- Sacred Yoga: www.sacredyoga.net

*Additional Sacred Living Movement mini-programs*

(Find these at www.sacredlivingmovement.com under "Retreats," "Classes," or "Sister Programs.")

- Sacred Year with Anni Daulter
- Sacred Self-Love
- Sacred Mother Blessing
- Sacred Crystals
- Sacred Healing Birth Trauma
- Sacred Scent
- Sacred Art
- Sacred Tarot
- Sacred Baby Feet (reflexology)
- Sacred Scent for Birth-Workers
- Sacred Blood Mysteries
- Sacred Medicine Cabinet
- Sacred Moon Mysteries
- Sacred Detox
- Sacred Belly Bind
- Sacred Tea
- Sacred Birth Dance
- Sacred Sisterhood Circles
- Sacred Mentor
- Sacred Book Intentions
- Sacred V-Steams
- Sacred Red Drum
- Sacred Elements
- Sacred Chakra
- Awakening the Heart
- Sacred Wild Woman
- Celtic Wheel

*International Sacred Living Movement websites:*

· Sacred Living Movement Canada: www.sacredlivingcanada.com
· Sacred Living Movement UK: www.sacredlivinguk.com

## *Some of our favorite places to buy herbs and flower essences*

**Golden Poppy Herbal Apothecary and Clinic**—your source in Fort Collins for herbs, teas, tinctures, essential oils, body care, nutrition, and more. Herbalist Sarah Josey contributed several recipes to this book, and is a wonderful resource if you have any questions or would like to buy herbs and remedies.

> 212 S. Mason St., Fort Collins, CO 80524, or 970-682-4373
> www.GoldenPoppyHerbs.com

**Soul Tree Essences**—Jessica Booth and Jessica Smithson co-create this beautiful line of flower and gem essences.

> www.thejessrose.com *in the USA*
> www.mamababywise.co.uk *in the U.K./Europe*

**Mountain Rose Herbs**—another ethical place to buy dried herbs in the USA.

> PO Box 50220, Eugene, OR 97405,
> or (toll-free) 1-800-879-3337
> www.mountainroseherbs.com

**Healing Waters**—an online store offering a huge range of flower and gem essences.

> www.essencesonline.com

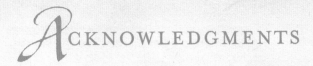

# ACKNOWLEDGMENTS

*From Anni Daulter*

Special thanks to everyone involved at North Atlantic Books: Tim, for saying yes to this sacred journey; Vanessa and Emily, for your dedication to the book; and Susan, for taking such a big chance on us. To all of the incredible photographers, particularly Heidi Marie, who put their work forward in this book with openness and love, this book would not be the same without you.

To Jessica Booth and Jessica Smithson, whom I met in the middle of the woods in Wales, where real faeries live and flowers and plants literally speak their magic. I could not be more blessed to have traveled across the seas to find you both, and you have inspired me, supported me and loved me through many twists and turns on this journey. Thank you. We have come a long way since Cae Mabon, and I am excited to see how we continue to unfold our visions together.

I must thank my sacred babies and my husband, Tim. You all teach me to be the best version of myself, and for that I am forever grateful. I love you all more than there are stars in the sky.

To my sisterhood of women who support me and the Sacred Living Movement, you know who you are, thank you. I love you all to the moon and back. To my music guru for all of your inspiration.

Lastly, but not least, thank you to my own mother, who raised me with such care of heart and soul and to my mother-in-law, Bonnie Walter, and my father-in-law, Dan Walter, for the never ending support you have shown me over the years. I love you all.

## From Jessica Booth

I'd like to thank everyone at North Atlantic Books, and all of the wonderful photographers, especially Heidi Marie and Megan Kibling, who shaped this book with such care and passion.

To Sarah Josey, Radha Schwaller, and all the others who generously shared recipes with us, I bow now in gratitude for your open hearts and knowledge. On this note, I honor the wisdom-keepers from around the world who held this medicine safe. I hope that we have shared your healing beauty with care and respect.

To Anni Daulter, thank you so much for your support, generosity, and collaboration. Meeting you and working with you has been life-changing in the most exciting ways.

To Jessica Smithson, what a wild ride since Cae Mabon, hey? I'm honored to be on this path with you.

To my family, thank you so much for all the careful nurturing of my gentle soul. Leigh, Eden, and Rai, you mean everything to me. Thank you to Andrew and Dad for your humor, heart, and wisdom. And thank you to my in-loves, Joyce and Kenny, for all your support.

To all my sacred sisters all over the world, especially in the Sacred Living Movement, thank you for holding me up, laughing with me, crying with me, and inspiring me all the time with your magic and love.

Finally, I'd like to thank the strong women in my family—my mom, Sherri, my grandmother, Barbara, my aunt Debra, my sister Alexis, and my cousin Katherine—who are healers, teachers, and wisdom-keepers in their own ways. You built a strong path for me to follow, and I am honored and privileged to be walking it with you. Thank you for showing me how it is done. I love you.

## From Jessica Smithson

I would like to start with a big, giant, special "thank you" to Anni Daulter for helping me see my gifts and be confident enough to share them with the world. From this my life is forever changed.

To Jessica Booth, my partner in so many amazing adventures, it's a joy to work with you. I am glad the universe brought us together.

Many thanks to North Atlantic Books for your trust and confidence in us.

To Christopher Penczak, ALisa Starkweather and Sue Jamison, your wisdom and knowledge has shaped my soul, and I am forever grateful.

I would like to thank so many people by name, but due to limited space let me just say that if you are in my life, I am learning from you, and appreciative of your medicine.

Lastly, to my mother, Deborah King, who would be so proud of me for being a part of this amazing collaboration—thank you, Mom, for being totally amazing and inspiring, and for showing me how it's done. I love you, and this book is for you.

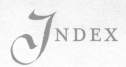

# INDEX

hydration, 70–71, 137
"hygiene hypothesis," 92

## I

"I Am Light," 392
"I am the Black Gold of The Sun," 184
Ice Pops, 162
imagination, 50
immunity
    ointment, 232–233
    strengthening, 230–231
incense, 140–141
inflammation, 65, 82–83, 136
infused oils, 52–53
ingredients list, 4
inner-smile meditation, 159
insomnia, 318
integration and release, 37
intentions, setting, 25
intestinal health, 282–283
intimacy and sex, talking about, 149

## J

Jeweled Rice, 51–52
Josey, Sarah, 41, 128, 181
journal. See wellness journal
joy, 159

## K

Kaur, Bachan, 30
Keep-It-Real Spritz, 151–152
ki, 104
Kidney I acupressure point, 252
kombucha, 283–284
kvass, 286–287

## L

labyrinth, walking, 288
"lack challenge," 223
Lakshmi Meditation, 225
laughter therapy, 158–159
Lavender and Rose Comfort Pillow, 378
lavender-infused oil, 52–53

LDL cholesterol, 198
lemon
    balm, 319
    and rosemary salt, 328
life-force, 104–105
Limitless Essence, 391–392
Lip Balm, 183
liquor, reducing, 36
listening empathetically, 308
lists
    equipment, 3
    ingredients, 4
liver cleanse, 36, 376
Love Honey, 139–140
Love Potion, 128–129
love vs. fear, 386–387
lung, 104
lungs inspiring health, 326
lutein, 118
lycopene, 48
lymphocytes, 230

## M

magic, 105–106
magnesium, 359
mandala design, using for yantra,
    27–28
mango body butter, 172–173
manipura, 150
Marigold Tea, 298–299
masks, playful feeling, 161
massage
    belly, 288
    oil, 82
    self, 171–172
Master's Tonic, 201–202
McKennitt, Loreena, 331
medicine
    "cosmic-orbit," 309–310
    food as, 14
    gratitude as, 364
    pleasure as, 126
    story and word, 294–295

air, earth, and fire, 296
dew-washing, 72
flavoring, 73
and hydration, 70–71
memory, 71–72
Sacred Bathing, 72
Weleda Rose Oil, 120
well-being, spiritual application, 13
wellness journal
accomplishment, 185–187
affirmations, 30–33
Beginner's Mind, 393–395
beginning, 12–13
bliss contemplation, 322–323
clean energy, 277–279
comfort foods, 352–353
connecting with senses, 100–101
cycles of life, 342–343
describing your glow, 176–177
dreams, 66–67, 204–205
empathetic listening, 314–315
follow your heart, 143–145
gratitude, 226–227, 370–371
guardian angel, 194–195
inner teen spirit, 153–155
integration and release, 43–45
life changes, 66–67
living without limits, 393–395
love letter to self, 87–89
magic, 110–111
moon cycle, 381–383
nourishment, 55–57
nurturing, 255–257
path of healing, 289–291
personal growth, 393–395
planning for year ahead, 332–333
playing, 163–165
pleasure, 132–133
positive changes, 20–21
reflections on balance, 20–21
rituals, 265–267
self-care, 245–247
senses, 121–123

sleep tracking, 360–361
spells, 300–301
spices, 204–205
thoughts, 66–67
transitions, 216–217
transmuting base metals, 204–205
water and quenching thirst, 75–77
wellness practices, 236–237
yantra meditation picture, 30–33
Whipped Mango Body Butter, 172–173
white chestnut flower essence, 319
white-colored foods, eating, 49
wild adventure, 93
wild heart, 93. *See also* heart
wildcrafting, best practices, 2
Wings and Prayers Ceremony, 193. *See also* praying and blessing
winter, qualities of, 306
wisdom potion, 191–192
wise one, becoming, 337
word and story medicine, 294–295
worry and overthinking, 210–211. *See also* anxiety

### ℋ

*Xiao Yao San,* 307–308

### Y

*yab-yum* tantric pose, 128
yantra, coloring, 27
yellow/orange-colored foods, eating, 49
Yoga Nidra, 357
Yoni Steam, 378–380
Yule Log Ceremony, 328–331

# 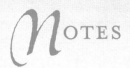OTES

1   Pollan, Michael, *In Defense of Food* (New York: Penguin Press, 2008).

2   Edelson, M., "Take two carrots and call me in the morning," *Hopkins Medicine* online edition (Winter 2010), www.hopkinsmedicine.org/hmn/w10 /feature2.cfm

3   Te Morenga, L., S. Mallard, and J. Mann, "Dietary sugars and body weight: systematic review and meta-analyses of randomised controlled trials and cohort studies," *British Medical Journal* (2013), www.bmj.com /content/346/bmj.e7492

4   Bennett, Connie and Stephen Sinatra. *Sugar Shock* (Berkeley, 2006).

5   Mesnage, R., N. Defarge, J. Spiroux de Vendomois, and G.-E. Seralini, "Major Pesticides Are More Toxic to Human Cells Than Their Declared Active Principles," BioMed Research International, vol. 2014, article ID 179691 (France, Feb 26, 2014), http://dx.doi.org/10.1155/2014/179691

6   Smith, Rick and Bruce Lourie, *Slow Death by Rubber Duck: How the Toxic Chemicals in Our Life Affect Our Health* (Toronto: Vintage Canada, Apr 2010).

7   Klein, A.V. and H. Kiat, "Detox diets for toxin elimination and weight management: a critical review of the evidence," *Journal of Human Nutrition and Dietetics* 28, no. 6 (Dec 18, 2014): 675–86, doi: 10.1111/jhn

8   International Food Information Council, "Eat a Rainbow: Functional Foods and Their Colorful Components," www.foodinsight.org /Eat_a_Rainbow_Functional_Foods_and_Their_Colorful_Components

9   Schaeffer, J., "Color Me Healthy—Eating a Rainbow of Benefits," *Today's Dietician* 10, no. 11 (Nov 2008): 34.

10  Lipton, Bruce, *The Biology of Belief: Unleashing the Power of Consciousness, Matter and Miracles* (Carlsbad: Mountain of Love, 2005).

11  Cowan, Eliot, *Plant Spirit Medicine* (Columbus, NC: Swan Raven, 1995 and Boulder, CO: Sounds True, Inc. 2014).

12  Buhner, Stephen Harrod, *The Secret Teachings of Plants: The Intelligence of the Heart in Direct Perception of Nature* (Rochester, VT: Bear and Company, 2004).

13  Shoba, G. et al., "Influence of piperine on the pharmacokinetics of curcumin in animals and human volunteers," *Planta Medica* 64, no. 4 (May 1998): 353–6.

14  Ody, Penelope, *Simple Healing with Herbs* (London: Chancellor Press, 2001): 51.

15  *op. cit.,* 65.

16  *op. cit.,* 67.

17  St. John Ambulance, "The Primary Survey," www.sja.org.uk/sja/first-aid-advice/what-to-do-as-a-first-aider/how-to-assess-a-casualty/the-primary-survey.aspx

18  http://blogs.redcross.org.uk/first-aid/2009/11/dr-abc-the-doctor-of-first-aid/

19  Dispenza, Dr. Joe, *You Are the Placebo: Making Your Mind Matter* (Carlsbad, CA: Hay House, Inc., Apr 2014).

20  Popkin, B., K. D'Anci, and I. Rosenberg, "Water Hydration and Health," *Nutrition Reviews* 68, no. 8 (Aug 2010): 439–458.

21  Radin, Dean, Nancy Lund, Masaru Emoto, and Takashige Kizu, "Effects of Distant Intention on Water Crystal Formation," *Journal of Scientific Exploration 22, no. 4* (2008).

22  Mohanta, Mahesh Prasad, "Growing Pains: Practitioner's Dilemma," *Indian Pediatrics* 51, no. 5 (May 2014): 379–383.

23  Morandi, Grazia et al., "Significant association among growing pains, vitamin D supplementation and bone mineral status: result from a pilot cohort study," The Japanese Society for Bone and Mineral Research (15 Mar 2014).

24  Alcantara, Joe and James Davis, "The chiropractic care of children with 'growing pains': a case series and systematic review of literature," *Complementary Therapies in Clinical Practice* 17, no. 1 (Feb 2011): 28–32.

25  Scarpa, Antonia and Antonio Guerci, "Various uses of the castor oil plant (*Ricinus communis L.*): a review," *Journal of Ethnopharmacology* 5, no. 2 (Mar 1982): 117–137.

26  Wold, A.E., "The hygiene hypothesis revised: is the rising frequency of allergy due to changes in the intestinal flora?" *Allergy* 53, suppl. 46 (1998): 20–25.

27  Azad, Meghan et al., "Infant gut microbiota and the hygiene hypothesis of allergic disease: impact of household pets and siblings on microbiota composition and diversity," *Allergy, Asthma and Clinical Immunology* 9 (2013): 15.

28 Dicksved, J. et al.: "Molecular fingerprinting of the fecal microbiota of children raised according to different lifestyles," *Applied and Environmental Microbiology* 73 (2007): 2,284–2,289.

29 Lowry, C.A. et al., "Identification of an immune-responsive mesolimbocortical serotonergic system: Potential role in regulation of emotional behavior," *Neuroscience* 146, no. 2 (May 2007): 756–772.

30 Faass, Nancy, "The Healing Powers of Wild Chaga," interview with Cass Ingram, MD, *Price-Pottenger Journal of Health and Healing* 35, no. 4 (Winter 2011–12).

31 Kahlos, K., L. Kangas, and R. Hiltunen, "Antitumor activity of some compounds and fractions from an n-hexane extract of Inonotus obliquus in vitro," *Acta Pharmaceutica Fennica* 96 (1987): 33–40.

32 Burczyk, J. et al., "Antimitotic activity of aqueous extracts of *Inonotus obliquus*," *Bollettino Chimico Farmaceutico (Boll Chim Farm)* 135 (1996): 306–9 [Medline].

33 Nilsson, Eric E. and Michael K. Skinner, "Environmentally induced epigenetic transgenerational inheritance of disease susceptibility," *Translational Research* 165, no. 1 (Jan 2015): 12–17.

34 Sassoli de Bianchi, M., "The Observer Effect," *Foundations of Science* 18 (2013): 213–243, arXiv:1109.3536

35 Lipton, Bruce, "The Wisdom in Your Cells" (Jun 2012), https://www.brucelipton.com/resource/article/the-wisdom-your-cells

36 "The Root Chakra: Muladhara," www.chopra.com/ccl/the-root-chakra-muladhara

37 The Dana Foundation, "The Senses: A Primer" (Sep 2013), www.brainfacts.org/sensing-thinking-behaving/senses-and-perception/articles/2013/the-senses-a-primer-part-i/

38 Kringelbach, Morten L. et al., "The Functional Neuroanatomy of Pleasure and Happiness," *Discovery Medicine* 9, no. 49 (Jun 2010): 579–587.

39 Ward, Devi, "Tantra Is Medicine" (2015), http://authentictantra.com/tantra-is-medicine/

40 Wauters, Ambika, *The Book of Chakras: Discover the Hidden Forces Within You* (Hauppauge, NY: Barron's Educational Series, Apr 2002).

41 Sandmaier, Marian, "Your Guide to a Healthy Heart," National Institute of Health's National Heart, Blood and Lung Institute (Dec 2005), https://www.nhlbi.nih.gov/files/docs/public/heart/healthyheart.pdf

42 Wauters, Ambika. *The Book of Chakras: Discover the Hidden Forces Within You* (Hauppauge, NY: Barron's Educational Series, Apr 2002).

43 Strean, William, "Laughter Prescription," *Canadian Family Physician* 55, no. 10 (Oct 2009): 965–967.

44  Cogan, R. et al., "Effects of Laughter and Relaxation on Discomfort Thresholds," *Journal of Behavioral Medicine* 10, no. 2 (1987): 139–144.

45  National Institute of Health's National Center for Complementary and Integrative Health, "Omega-3 Supplements in Depth," Pub. #D482 (Jul 2009), https://nccih.nih.gov/health/omega3/introduction.htm

46  Nair, Rathish and Arun Maseeh, "Vitamin D: the "Sunshine Vitamin," *Journal of Pharmacology and Pharmacotherapeutics* 3, no. 2 (Apr–Jun 2012): 118–126.

47  Andrade, Chittaranjan and Rajiv Radhakrishnan, "Prayer and healing: A medical and scientific perspective on randomized controlled trials," *Indian Journal of Psychiatry* 51, no. 4 (Oct–Dec 2009): 247–253.

48  "The Crown Chakra: Sahaswara," www.chopra.com/ccl/connect-to-the -divine-with-the-seventh-chakra

49  Kawatra, Pallavi and Rathai Rajagopalan, "Cinnamon: Mystic Powers of a Minute Ingredient," *Pharmacognosy Research* 7, no. 5, suppl. 1 (Jun 2015): S1–S6

50  Bode, Ann M. and Zigang Dong, "The Amazing and Mighty Ginger," in *Herbal Medicine: Biomolecular and Clinical Aspects*, 2nd ed. (Taylor and Francis Group, LLC, 2011).

51  Ahuja, Kiran D. et al., "Effects of Chili Consumption on Postprandial Glucose, Insulin and Energy Metabolism," *American Journal of Clinical Nutrition* 84, no. 1 (Jul 2006): 63–69.

52  Garcia, Charles R., "Garlic and Cayenne," California School of Traditional Hispanic Herbalism, www.hispanicherbs.com/articles.html

53  Bayan, Leyla et al., "Garlic: A Review of Potential Therapeutic Effects," *Avicenna Journal of Phytomedicine* 4, no. 1 (Jan–Feb 2014): 1–14.

54  Honan, Daniel, "Neuroplasticity: You Can Teach an Old Brain New Tricks," http://bigthink.com/think-tank/brain-exercise

55  S. Chetty et al., "Stress and glucocorticoids promote oligodendrogenesis in the adult hippocampus," *Molecular Psychiatry* 19 (Dec 2014): 1,275–1,283.

56  Dyall, Simon C., "Long-chain omega-3 fatty acids and the brain: a review of the independent and shared effects of EPA, DPA and DHA," *Frontiers in Aging Neuroscience* 7 (2015): 52.

57  Chacko, Sabu M. et al., "Beneficial effects of green tea: a literature review," *Chinese Medicine* 5 (2010): 13.

58  Burton, Neel, "How To Improve Your Concentration and Memory," *Psychology Today* (Jan 2013), https://www.psychologytoday.com/blog /hide-and-seek/201301/how-improve-your-concentration-and-memory

59  Nemours Foundation, "Immune System," http://kidshealth.org/en /parents/immune.html

60 Harvard Health Publications, "How to Boost Your Immune System," www.health.harvard.edu/staying-healthy /how-to-boost-your-immune-system

61 Wauters, Ambika, *The Book of Chakras: Discover the Hidden Forces Within You* (Hauppauge, NY: Barron's Educational Series, April, 2002).

62 "Elderberry *(Sambucus nigra)*: Health Benefits of Elderberries," www .herbwisdom.com/herb-elderberry.html

63 Bjelakovic, Goran et al., "Antioxidant Supplements and Mortality," Current Opinion in *Clinical Nutrition and Metabolic Care* 17, no. 1 (Jan 2014): 40–44.

64 Carlsen, Monica H. et al., "The total antioxidant content of more than 3100 foods, beverages, spices, herbs and supplements used worldwide," *Nutrition Journal* 9 (2010): 3.

65 Schneiderman, Neil et al., "Stress and Health: Psychological, Behavioral and Biological Determinants," *Annual Review of Clinical Psychology* 1 (2005): 607–628.

66 Nordqvist, Christian, "What is Stress? How to Deal with Stress," *Medical News Today* (Dec 2015), www.medicalnewstoday.com/articles/145855.php

67 Beresford-Cooke, Carola, *Shiatsu Theory and Practice*, 3rd ed. (London: Singing Dragon, Mar 2016).

68 Pope, Alexandra, *The Wild Genie: the Healing Power of Menstruation* (London: New Generation Publishing, 2014).

69 Zhang, Yu-Jie, "Impacts of Gut Bacteria on Human Health and Diseases," *International Journal of Molecular Sciences* 16, no. 4 (Apr 2015): 7,493–7,519.

70 Power, Susan E. et al., "Intestinal Microbiota, Diet and Health," *British Journal of Nutrition* 11, no. 03 (Feb 2014): 387–402.

71 March, Alan et al., "Sequence-based analysis of the bacterial and fungal compositions of multiple kombucha (tea fungus) samples," *Food Microbiology* 38 (Apr 2014): 171–178.

72 Kaufmann, Klaus, D.Sc., "Health Benefits of Drinking Kombucha Tea," *Mother Earth News* (Mar 17, 2014), www.motherearthnews.com /natural-health/herbal-remedies/health-benefits-of-drinking -kombucha-tea-ze0z1303zcalt.aspx

73 National Institute of Mental Health, "Depression" (rev. May 2016), https://www.nimh.nih.gov/health/topics/depression/index.shtml

74 Smith, Melinda et al., "Helping a Depressed Person" (Apr 2016), www .helpguide.org/articles/depression/helping-a-depressed-person.htm

75 Linde, Klaus et al., "St. John's wort for depression: Meta-analysis of randomised controlled trials," *The British Journal of Psychiatry* 186, no. 2 (Jan 2005): 99–107.

76  Butler, Lee and Karen Pilkington, "Chinese Herbal Medicine and Depression: The Research Evidence," *Evidence-Based Complementary and Alternative Medicine* (2013), http://dx.doi.org/10.1155/2013/739716

77  "*Xiao Yao San* (Rambling Powder, Free and Easy Wanderer)," https://www.sacredlotus.com/go/chinese-formulas/medicine/xiao-yao-san

78  Dillinger, Teresa et al., "Food of the Gods: Cure for Humanity? A Cultural History of the Medicinal and Ritual Use of Chocolate," *Journal of Nutrition* 130, no. 8 (Aug 1, 2000): 2,057S–2,072S.

79  Grieve, M., "Cacao," https://www.botanical.com/botanical/mgmh/c/cacao-02.html

80  Anxiety and Depression Association of America, "Tips to Manage Anxiety and Stress," www.adaa.org/tips-manage-anxiety-and-stress

81  University of Maryland Medical Center (rev Jun 2014), "Passionflower," umm.edu/health/medical/altmed/herb/passionflower

82  University of Maryland Medical Center (rev Jan 2015), "Lemon Balm," umm.edu/health/medical/altmed/herb/lemon-balm

83  Mayo Clinic, "Bone Health" (Jan 2015), www.Mayoclinic.org

84  Meremikwu, M.M. and A. Oyo-Ita, "Paracetemol for Treating Fever in Children," *Cochrane Library* (Apr 2003).

85  Meremikwu, M.M. and A. Oyo-Ita, "Physical Methods for Treating Fever in Children," *Cochrane Library* (Apr 2003).

86  Contie, Vicki et al., "Benefits of Slumber," *NIH News in Health* (Apr 2013), https://newsinhealth.nih.gov/issue/apr2013/feature1

87  Yoga Nidra Network, www.yoganidranetwork.org/downloads

88  Greater Good Science Center, "Expanding the Science and Practice of Gratitude," http://greatergood.berkeley.edu/expandinggratitude

89  Wauters, Ambika, *The Book of Chakras: Discover the Hidden Forces Within You* (Hauppauge, NY: Barron's Educational Series, Apr 2002).

# $\mathcal{A}$BOUT THE AUTHORS

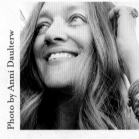

**ANNI DAULTER** is the author of *Sacred Pregnancy* (North Atlantic Books 2012), coauthor of *Sacred Motherhood* (North Atlantic Books 2016), and founder of the Sacred Living Movement. She travels the world leading retreats that inspire, uplift, and connect women in many areas of their lives. She trains birth-workers to lead Sacred Pregnancy classes, helps couples heal at Sacred Relationship retreats, empowers women at i am Sisterhood retreats, and brings moms and daughters together in celebration at Sacred Sweeties retreats. Anni has written six other books to inspire natural family living, and is an artist of the Beauty Way. She ventures a high-vibration lifestyle with her husband, Tim, and her four children, Zoë, Lotus Sunshine, Bodhi, and River.

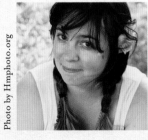

**JESSICA BOOTH** is a healer and writer, thriving in family community at Sweet Lovin' Ranch, California. She joined the Sacred Living Movement in 2014, and runs Sacred Essence and Sacred Fertility programs with Jessica Smithson. These classes and retreats foster a connection with nature, body, and spirit. Jessica is a priestess and a red-drum carrier with the Red Moon Mystery School. She supports people on their unique journeys through womanhood and health at all stages of their lives, using her background in several energy medicine modalities, naturopathic nutrition, and shiatsu. She believes in awakening the sleeping dreams, in caring for the tender buds of the soul, and most of all in living with love.

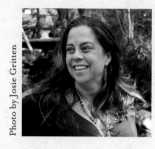

Photo by Josie Gritten

JESSICA SMITHSON is a creative kinesi-ologist, doula, and leader within the Sacred Living Movement. She has a background in energy medicine, Native American Medicine, and esoteric mystery teachings. She is a flow-er-essence practitioner and the cocreator of Soul Tree Essences, and loves spending time in nature. Jessica teaches the online classes Sacred Essence, Sacred Baby and Mother Blessing, Sacred Blood Mysteries, Sacred Fertility, and Mama's Sacred Medicine Cupboard. She also runs live retreats for Sacred Fertility, supporting couples with their fertility journeys and training fertility doulas to carry the work forward. She specializes in feeding people on many levels, from physical food to spiritual suste-nance, attempting to empower everyone she meets to find their own medicine.

# 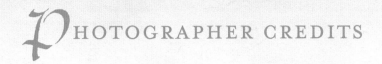PHOTOGRAPHER CREDITS

Firstly, we want to extend all of our heart-felt thank you to the primary photographer for *Sacred Medicine Cupboard*, Heidi Marie. Her dedication to this project was amazing, and her photography vision is her medicine to the world. Thank you, Heidi! The team that assisted Heidi, Little Oyster styling team (Anni Daulter + Jessica Booth) and extra help on the photo shoots, was the very lovely crew of Jessica Smithson, Sue Crowder, and Luna. We have deep gratitude for all the folks who came together to make this book look as beautiful as it does!

Many other photographers shared their beautiful visionary work with us to make *Sacred Medicine Cupboard* as stunning as it is. A special thanks to Megan Kibling-Elizondo, Trevor Mars of SoulMakes, Camilla Albano-Fotografia, The Visionary Photographic Art of Chanel Baran, Zipporah Lomax, Alicia D'Amico, Katy Leet and Lindsay Holt, and Tnah Louise.

**BOOK OPENER**
"Handprint," Tnah Louise

## SPRING

Spring opener photo: "Spring Energy," Soulmakes, www.soulmakes.com

**CHAPTER 1: THE DAWN**
Main photo: "Medicine Cupboard," Heidi Marie Wagstaff, Hmphoto.org, styling: Anni Daulter at Little Oyster; top photo: "Dawn Nature," Soulmakes, www.soulmakes.com; bottom photo: "Flower Essence," Heidi Marie Wagstaff,

Hmphoto.org, styling: Anni Daulter at Little Oyster; inside photo: "Cleaning Powder," Heidi Marie Wagstaff, Hmphoto.org, styling: Anni Daulter at Little Oyster

## CHAPTER 2: AWAKENING

Main photo: "Goddess," Camilla Albano-Fotografia, https://www.flickr .com/photos/camilla_albano; top Photo: "Rose Petal," Heidi Marie Wagstaff, Hmphoto.org, styling: Anni Daulter at Little Oyster; bottom photo: "Tea Mandala," Lindsay Holt of Altar and Leaf Apotheca, http://www .altarandleaf.com/; inside photo: "Yantra Drawing," Iris Kern-Foster, kernfoster.com

## CHAPTER 3: SPRING EQUINOX

Main photo: "Spring Goddess," Soulmakes, www.soulmakes.com; top photo: "Vinegar Rinse," Heidi Marie Wagstaff, Hmphoto.org, styling: Anni Daulter at Little Oyster; bottom photo: "Dry Brushing," Heidi Marie Wagstaff, Hmphoto.org, styling: Anni Daulter at Little Oyster; inside photo: "Coconut Shampoo," Corinne Laan, www.birthbliss.nl

## CHAPTER 4: THE BUD

Main photo: "Flower Curtain," Soulmakes, www.soulmakes.com; top photo: "Rainbow Veggies," Heidi Marie Wagstaff, Hmphoto.org, styling: Anni Daulter at Little Oyster; bottom photo: "Salve," Heidi Marie Wagstaff, Hmphoto.org, styling: Anni Daulter at Little Oyster; inside photo: "Rose Oil," Heidi Marie Wagstaff, Hmphoto.org, styling: Anni Daulter at Little Oyster

## CHAPTER 5: BLOSSOM

Main photo: "Flower Crown Goddess," Myrriah Raimbault, Peaceful Birth Haven, http://www.peacefulbirthhaven.com/; top photo: "Creek Flowers," Heidi Marie Wagstaff, Hmphoto.org, styling: Anni Daulter at Little Oyster; bottom photo: "Flower Board," Heidi Marie Wagstaff, Hmphoto.org, styling: Anni Daulter at Little Oyster; inside photo: "Essence Bottles," Heidi Marie Wagstaff, Hmphoto.org, styling: Anni Daulter at Little Oyster

## CHAPTER 6: RENEWAL

Main photo: "Dew Greens," Soulmakes, www.soulmakes.com; top photo: "Creek Cleanse," Megan Kibling-Elizondo, Nutmeg Photography, http://nutmegphotos.smugmug.com/; bottom photo: "Herb Bundle," Heidi Marie Wagstaff, Hmphoto.org, styling: Anni Daulter at Little Oyster; inside photo: "Flavored Herbal Water," Heidi Marie Wagstaff, Hmphoto.org, styling: Anni Daulter at Little Oyster

## CHAPTER 7: GROWTH

Main photo: "Green Goddess," Katy Leet, www.katyleetphotography.com; top photo: "Growth Balm," Heidi Marie Wagstaff, Hmphoto.org, styling: Anni Daulter at Little Oyster; bottom photo: "Free Herbs," Heidi Marie Wagstaff, Hmphoto.org, styling: Anni Daulter at Little Oyster; inside photo: "Soothe Me Oats," Heidi Marie Wagstaff, Hmphoto.org, styling: Anni Daulter at Little Oyster

## CHAPTER 8: THE WILD

Main photo: "Nature Goddess," The Visionary Photographic Art of Chanel Baran, www.ChanelBaran.com, Muse: Josie Walker, http://coloradomountainranch.com/; top photo: "Dirt Hands," Heidi Marie Wagstaff, Hmphoto.org, styling: Anni Daulter at Little Oyster; bottom photo: "Bug Bite Spritzer," Heidi Marie Wagstaff, Hmphoto.org, styling: Anni Daulter at Little Oyster; inside photo: "Chaga," Marnie Burkhart, Jazhart Studios Inc., marnie@jazhart.com, www.jazhart.com

## CHAPTER 9: MAGIC

Main photo: "Earth Goddess," Alicia D'Amico, pureemotionsphotography.com, Pure Emotions Photography; top photo: "Root Essence," Heidi Marie Wagstaff, Hmphoto.org, styling: Anni Daulter at Little Oyster; bottom photo: "Free to Be Me," Heidi Marie Wagstaff, Hmphoto.org, styling: Anni Daulter at Little Oyster; inside photo: "Crystal Essence," Heidi Marie Wagstaff, Hmphoto.org, styling: Anni Daulter at Little Oyster

# SUMMER

Summer opener photo: "Summer Flowers," Jane Ferrell, Jane in the Woods, www.janeinthewoods.com

## CHAPTER 10: MIDDAY

Main photo: stock photo; top photo: "Creek Feet," Heidi Marie Wagstaff, Hmphoto.org; bottom Photo: "Serenity Essence," Heidi Marie Wagstaff, Hmphoto.org, Styling: Anni Daulter at Little Oyster; inside photo: "Avocado Face Mask," Heidi Marie Wagstaff, Hmphoto.org, styling: Anni Daulter at Little Oyster

## CHAPTER 11: TANTRA

Main photo: "Flower Arms," Heidi Marie Wagstaff, Hmphoto.org, styling: Anni Daulter at Little Oyster; top photo: "Beet Lips," Heidi Marie Wagstaff, Hmphoto.org, styling: Anni Daulter at Little Oyster; bottom photo: "Potion," Heidi Marie Wagstaff, Hmphoto.org, styling: Anni Daulter at Little Oyster; inside photo: "Love Honey," Heidi Marie Wagstaff, Hmphoto.org, styling: Anni Daulter at Little Oyster

## CHAPTER 12: SUMMER SOLSTICE

Main photo: "Water Goddess," Sari Mattsson, http://www.sarimattsson.com/; top photo: "Bottles," Jane Ferrell, Jane in the Woods, www.janeinthewoods .com; bottom photo: "Self-Doubt Fire," Katy Leet, www.katyleetphotography .com; inside photo: "Dandy Essence," Heidi Marie Wagstaff, Hmphoto.org, styling: Anni Daulter at Little Oyster

## CHAPTER 13: THE FLOWER

Main photo: "Flowers on Board," Heidi Marie Wagstaff, Hmphoto.org, styling: Anni Daulter at Little Oyster; top photo: "Chocolate Face Masks," Tnah Louise, Bella Faccia Foto, bellafacciafoto.com; bottom photo: "Walking the Path," Heidi Marie Wagstaff, Hmphoto.org, styling: Anni Daulter at Little Oyster; inside photo: "Rose Water Clarity Wand," Heidi Marie Wagstaff, Hmphoto.org, styling: Anni Daulter at Little Oyster

## CHAPTER 14: PLAY

Main photo: "Erin Laughing," Megan Kibling-Elizondo, Nutmeg Photography, http://nutmegphotos.smugmug.com/; top photo: "Green Ice Pops," Heidi Marie Wagstaff, Hmphoto.org, styling: Anni Daulter at Little Oyster; bottom photo: "Bubbles," Heidi Marie Wagstaff, Hmphoto.org, styling: Anni Daulter at Little Oyster; inside photo: "Story Stones," Heidi Marie Wagstaff, Hmphoto .org, styling: Anni Daulter at Little Oyster, Story Stones by: Angie Falk

## CHAPTER 15: GLOW

Main photo: "Sacred Ayurveda Journal," Sari Mattsson, http://www.sarimattsson.com/; top photo: "Spices," Radha Schwaller, www.sacred-ayurveda.com; bottom photo: "Bath Bombs," Heidi Marie Wagstaff, Hmphoto.org, styling: Anni Daulter at Little Oyster; inside photo: "Whipped Body Butter," Heidi Marie Wagstaff, Hmphoto.org, styling: Anni Daulter at Little Oyster

## CHAPTER 16: THE SUN

Main photo: "The Rising Sun," Heidi Marie Wagstaff, Hmphoto.org, top photo: "Aloe," Heidi Marie Wagstaff, Hmphoto.org, styling: Anni Daulter at Little Oyster; bottom photo: "Lip Balm Pour," Heidi Marie Wagstaff, Hmphoto.org, styling: Anni Daulter at Little Oyster; inside photo: "Sunscreen," Heidi Marie Wagstaff, Hmphoto.org, styling: Anni Daulter at Little Oyster, Sunscreen Created by: Sarah Josey of Golden Poppy Herbal Apothecary

## CHAPTER 17: WINGS

Main photo: "Ceremonial Wings," Heidi Marie Wagstaff, Hmphoto.org, styling: Anni Daulter at Little Oyster; top photo: "Prayer Goddess," The Visionary Photographic Art of Chanel Baran, www.ChanelBaran.com, Muse: Josie Walker, http://coloradomountainranch.com/; bottom photo: "Potion," Heidi Marie Wagstaff, Hmphoto.org, styling: Anni Daulter at Little Oyster; inside photo: "Feather," Soulmakes, www.soulmakes.com

## CHAPTER 18: ALCHEMY

Main photo: "The Good Witch," Heidi Marie Wagstaff, Hmphoto.org, styling: Anni Daulter at Little Oyster; top photo: "Spices," Katy Leet, www.katyleetphotography.com; bottom photo: "Fire Cider," Heidi Marie Wagstaff, Hmphoto.org, styling: Anni Daulter at Little Oyster; inside photo: "Cayenne Balm," Heidi Marie Wagstaff, Hmphoto.org, styling: Anni Daulter at Little Oyster

# FALL

Fall Opener Photo: "Making Medicine," Heidi Marie Wagstaff, Hmphoto.org, styling: Anni Daulter at Little Oyster

## CHAPTER 19: TWILIGHT

Main photo: "Smudging," Zipporah Lomax, http://zipporahlomax.com/; top photo: "Rose Petal Herb Bundle," Heidi Marie Wagstaff, Hmphoto.org, styling: Anni Daulter at Little Oyster; bottom photo: "Journal," Heidi Marie Wagstaff, Hmphoto.org; inside photo: "Concentration Bites," Heidi Marie Wagstaff, Hmphoto.org, styling: Anni Daulter at Little Oyster

## CHAPTER 20: ABUNDANCE

Main photo: "Trust," Zipporah Lomax, http://zipporahlomax.com/; top photo: "Release Lack," Anni Daulter, styling: Anni Daulter at Little Oyster; bottom photo: "Peru Ceremony," The Visionary Photographic Art of Chanel Baran, www.ChanelBaran.com, Fire Mane www.pachartakiyperutours.com; inside photo: "Abundance Oil," Anni Daulter photo + styling, Abundance Oil created by Dawn McCorry

## CHAPTER 21: AUTUMN EQUINOX

Main photo: "Elderberry Syrup," Heidi Marie Wagstaff, Hmphoto.org, styling: Anni Daulter at Little Oyster; top photo: "Hands," Megan Kibling--Elizondo, Nutmeg Photography, http://nutmegphotos.smugmug.com/; bottom photo: "Kylie in Nature," Heidi Marie Wagstaff, Hmphoto.org, styling: Anni Daulter at Little Oyster; inside photo: "Gratitude Tree," Heidi Marie Wagstaff, Hmphoto.org, styling: Anni Daulter at Little Oyster

## CHAPTER 22: THE FRUIT

Main photo: "Pom Shot," Heidi Marie Wagstaff, Hmphoto.org, styling: Anni Daulter at Little Oyster; top photo: "YES," Zipporah Lomax, http://zipporahlomax.com/; bottom photo: "Red Drink," Heidi Marie Wagstaff, Hmphoto.org, styling: Anni Daulter at Little Oyster; inside photo: "Pom Sugar Scrub," Heidi Marie Wagstaff, Hmphoto.org, styling: Anni Daulter at Little Oyster

## CHAPTER 23: NURTURE

Main photo: "Tonic," Heidi Marie Wagstaff, Hmphoto.org, styling: Anni Daulter at Little Oyster; top photo: "Soothing Headache Rollarball," Heidi Marie Wagstaff, Hmphoto.org, styling: Anni Daulter at Little Oyster; bottom photo: stock photo; inside photo: "Tummy Tea," Heidi Marie Wagstaff, Hmphoto.org, styling: Anni Daulter at Little Oyster

## CHAPTER 24: RITE

Main photo: "Warrior Oil," Heidi Marie Wagstaff, Hmphoto.org, styling: Anni Daulter at Little Oyster; top photo: "Luna Ceremony," Myrriah Raimbault, Peaceful Birth Haven, http://www.peacefulbirthhaven.com/; bottom photo: "Ceremony Candles," Myrriah Raimbault, Peaceful Birth Haven, http://www.peacefulbirthhaven.com/; inside photo: "Drum," Megan Kibling-Elizondo, Nutmeg Photography, http://nutmegphotos.smugmug.com/

## CHAPTER 25: GATHER

Main photo: "Gather Sticks," Heidi Marie Wagstaff, Hmphoto.org, styling: Anni Daulter at Little Oyster; top photo: "Neti Pot," Heidi Marie Wagstaff, Hmphoto.org, styling: Anni Daulter at Little Oyster; bottom photo: "Stone Soup," Heidi Marie Wagstaff, Hmphoto.org, styling: Anni Daulter at Little Oyster; inside photo: "Onion," Heidi Marie Wagstaff, Hmphoto.org, styling: Anni Daulter at Little Oyster

## CHAPTER 26: THE LABYRINTH

Main photo: "Kvass," Heidi Marie Wagstaff, Hmphoto.org, styling: Anni Daulter at Little Oyster; top photo: "Bitters," Heidi Marie Wagstaff, Hmphoto.org, styling: Anni Daulter at Little Oyster; bottom photo: "Labyrinth," Kiera Lillesve, www.kieralillesvefoto.com; inside photo: "Fermented," Heidi Marie Wagstaff, Hmphoto.org, styling: Anni Daulter at Little Oyster

## CHAPTER 27: SPELL

Main photo: "Bow Now," The Visionary Photographic Art of Chanel Baran, www.ChanelBaran.com, Fire Mane, www.pachartakiyperutours.com; "Clarity," Zipporah Lomax, http://zipporahlomax.com/; bottom photo: "Herb Bowl," Heidi Marie Wagstaff, Hmphoto.org, styling: Anni Daulter at Little Oyster; inside photo: "Black Salt," Heidi Marie Wagstaff, Hmphoto.org, styling: Anni Daulter at Little Oyster

# WINTER

Winter opener photo: "Holiday Spirit," Soulmakes, www.soulmakes.com

## CHAPTER 28: MIDNIGHT

Main photo: stock photo; top photo: "I Am Enough," Heidi Marie Wagstaff, Hmphoto.org; bottom photo: "Chocolate," Heidi Marie Wagstaff, Hmphoto.org, styling: Anni Daulter at Little Oyster; inside photo: "Kitchen Witch," Heidi Marie Wagstaff, Hmphoto.org, styling: Anni Daulter at Little Oyster

## CHAPTER 29: CONTEMPLATION

Main photo: stock photo; top photo: "Surrender," The Visionary Photographic Art of Chanel Baran, www.ChanelBaran.com, Muse: Josie Walker, http://coloradomountainranch.com/; bottom photo: "White Iris Essence," Heidi Marie Wagstaff, Hmphoto.org, styling: Anni Daulter at Little Oyster; inside photo: "Peace Tea," Heidi Marie Wagstaff, Hmphoto.org, Styling: Anni Daulter at Little Oyster

## CHAPTER 30: WINTER SOLSTICE

Main photo: stock photo; top photo: "The Gift," Heidi Marie Wagstaff, Hmphoto.org, styling: Anni Daulter at Little Oyster; bottom photo: "Herbal Infused Salts," Heidi Marie Wagstaff, Hmphoto.org, styling: Anni Daulter at Little Oyster; inside photo: "Pine + Holly Blessing Water," Heidi Marie Wagstaff, Hmphoto.org, styling: Anni Daulter at Little Oyster

## CHAPTER 31: THE SEED

Main photo: "Virility Tonic," Heidi Marie Wagstaff, Hmphoto.org, styling: Anni Daulter at Little Oyster; top photo: "Ancestors," Soulmakes, www.soulmakes.com; bottom Photo: "Set Up Goodies," Heidi Marie Wagstaff, Hmphoto.org, styling: Anni Daulter at Little Oyster; inside photo: "Crystal Grid," Heidi Marie Wagstaff, Hmphoto.org, styling: Anni Daulter + Jessica Smithson at Little Oyster

## CHAPTER 32: NOURISH

Main photo: "Mushrroms + Veggies Broth," Heidi Marie Wagstaff, Hmphoto.org, styling: Anni Daulter at Little Oyster; top photo: "Tea Cups," Katy Leet, www.katyleetphotography.com; bottom photo: "Mixing Herbs with Hands," Katy Leet, www.katyleetphotography.com; inside photo: "Bone Broth," Anni Daulter, Styling: Anni Daulter at Little Oyster

## CHAPTER 33: REST

Main photo: "Yoga Nidra," Heidi Marie Wagstaff, Hmphoto.org, styling: Anni Daulter at Little Oyster; top photo: "Dreamy Stars," Heidi Marie Wagstaff, Hmphoto.org, styling: Anni Daulter at Little Oyster; bottom photo: "Warm Milk," Heidi Marie Wagstaff, Hmphoto.org, Styling: Anni Daulter at Little Oyster; inside photo: "Herbal Bath Salts," Heidi Marie Wagstaff, Hmphoto.org, styling: Anni Daulter at Little Oyster

## CHAPTER 34: GRATITUDE

Main photo: "Prayers," Megan Kibling-Elizondo, Nutmeg Photography, http://nutmegphotos.smugmug.com, Muse: Sarah Josey; top photo: "Gratitude Stones," Heidi Marie Wagstaff, Hmphoto.org, styling: Anni Daulter at Little Oyster; bottom photo: "Heart Shape Bath Bombs," Heidi Marie Wagstaff, Hmphoto.org, styling: Anni Daulter at Little Oyster; inside photo: "Earth Feet," Heidi Marie Wagstaff, Hmphoto.org, styling: Anni Daulter at Little Oyster

## CHAPTER 35: THE MOON

Main photo: stock photo; top photo: stock photo; bottom photo: "Honoring Moontime," The Visionary Photographic Art of Chanel Baran, www.ChanelBaran.com, Muse: Womb Illumination by Divine Flow, http://wombillumination.com; inside photo: "Roses + Lavendar Pillow Herbs," Heidi Marie Wagstaff, Hmphoto.org, styling: Anni Daulter at Little Oyster

## CHAPTER 36: CONJURE

Main photo: "Conjuring Goddess," The Visionary Photographic Art of Chanel Baran, www.ChanelBaran.com, Muse: Jaya Nirvana, https://www.instagram.com/cosmic.weaver/; top photo: "Inspired Cards," Zipporah Lomax, http://zipporahlomax.com/; bottom photo: "Salt Bowl," Tnah Louise, Bella Faccia Foto, bellafacciafoto.com; inside photo: "Citrine Essence," Heidi Marie Wagstaff, Hmphoto.org, styling: Anni Daulter at Little Oyster

# TITLES BY ANNI DAULTER
*available from North Atlantic Books*

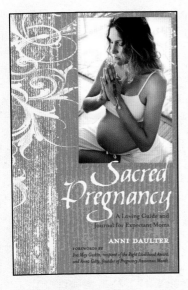

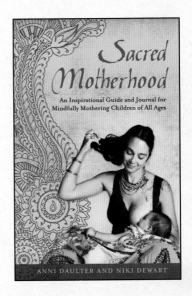

*Sacred Pregnancy*
978-1-58394-444-8

*Sacred Motherhood*
978-1-62317-004-2

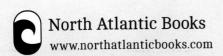

**North Atlantic Books**
www.northatlanticbooks.com

North Atlantic Books is an independent, nonprofit publisher committed to a bold exploration of the relationships between mind, body, spirit, and nature.